DUAL ENERGY X-RAY ABSORPTIOMETRY

Edited by **Abdellah El Maghraoui**

Dual Energy X-Ray Absorptiometry
Edited by Abdellah El Maghraoui

Published by InTech

Janeza Trdine 9, 51000 Rijeka, Croatia

Publishing Process Manager Dejan Grgur

Technical Editor Teodora Smiljanic

Cover Designer InTech Design Team

Additional hard copies can be obtained from orders@intechopen.com

Dual Energy X-Ray Absorptiometry, Edited by Abdellah El Maghraoui
p. cm.
ISBN 978-953-307-877-9

For EU product safety concerns:
IN TECH d.o.o., Prolaz Marije Krucifikse Kozulić 3, 51000 Rijeka, Croatia,
info@intechopen.com or visit our website at intechopen.com.

Meet the editor

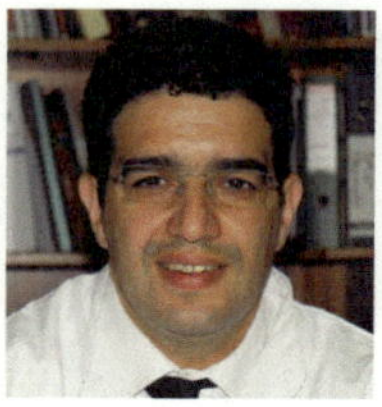

Prof. El Maghraoui was born in 1969, and is currently a Professor of Rheumatology at the Rabat Medicine and Pharmacy University. He is also the head of the Rheumatology Department, Military Hospital Mohammed V, Rabat, Morocco, and the vice president of the Moroccan Society of Rheumatology. He graduated from the Rabat Medicine and Pharmacy University, and received diplomas in Podology from the Paris V University, in Muscular Ultrasound from the Paris VI University, and in Methodology of Clinical Research from the Bordeaux University. Prof. El Maghraoui has authored more than 90 PubMed indexed articles, and has published a book titled L'ostéoporose in 2010. He is also the founder, designer and Webmaster of www.rhumato.info, a website for public health professionals, dedicated to rheumatology.

Contents

Preface XI

Part 1 Bone Mineral Density 1

Chapter 1 **Interpreting a DXA Scan in Clinical Practice 3**
Abdellah El Maghraoui

Chapter 2 **Monitoring DXA Measurement in Clinical Practice 19**
Abdellah El Maghraoui

Chapter 3 **Bone Loss and Seasonal Variation in Serial DXA Densitometry – A Population-Based Study 29**
Joonas Sirola, Toni Rikkonen, Risto Honkanen, Jukka S. Jurvelin, Marjo Tuppurainen and Heikki Kröger

Part 2 Body Composition 43

Chapter 4 **The Validity of Body Composition Measurement Using Dual Energy X-Ray Absorptiometry for Estimating Resting Energy Expenditure 45**
Chiyoko Usui, Motoko Taguchi, Kazuko Ishikawa-Takata and Mitsuru Higuchi

Chapter 5 **Dxa as a Tool for the Assessment of Morphological Asymmetry in Athletes 59**
Magdalena Krzykała

Chapter 6 **Body Composition in Disabilities of Central Nervous System 75**
Yannis Dionyssiotis

Part 3 Miscellaneous 95

Chapter 7 **Internal Design of the Dry Human Ulna by DXA 97**
S. Aguado-Henche, A. Bosch-Martín, P. Spottorno-Rubio and R. Rodríguez-Torres

Chapter 8 ***Ex Vivo* and *In Vivo* Assessment of Vertebral Strength and Vertebral Fracture Risk Assessed by Dual Energy X-Ray Absorptiometry 105**
Kazuhiro Imai

Chapter 9 **Dietary Protein and Bone Health 121**
Anne Blais, Emilien Rouy and Daniel Tomé

Preface

Dual-energy x-ray absorptiometry (DXA) is now recognized as the reference method to measure bone mineral density (BMD) with acceptable accuracy errors, good precision and reproducibility. The World Health Organization (WHO) has established DXA as the best densitometric technique for assessing BMD in postmenopausal women and has based the definitions of osteopenia and osteoporosis on its results. DXA allows accurate diagnosis of osteoporosis, estimation of fracture risk and monitoring of patients undergoing treatment. Correct performance of BMD measurements using DXA requires rigorous attention to detail in positioning and analysis. Performing DXA studies incorrectly can lead to major mistakes in diagnosis and therapy. Measurement error must be considered when evaluating serial assessments. A clear understanding of the interpretation of serial measurements and the statistical principles impacting upon their interpretation is necessary to determine whether a change is real and not simply random fluctuation. Moreover, it is important to keep in mind that fracture-protection benefit may be realized before BMD gains are detected. Physicians interested in osteoporosis management, even if not directly involved in the performance and interpretation of DXA, should be familiar with the principles of DXA to minimize serious errors and allow proper use of bone densitometry.

Additional features of DXA include measurement of BMD at multiple skeletal sites, vertebral fracture assessment (also called vertebral morphometry) using evaluation of vertebral heights with a special software to determine vertebral body dimensions, body composition assessment including bone mineral content, fat mass and lean soft tissue mass of the whole body and the segments.

This book contains reviews and original studies about DXA and many different uses in clinical practice (diagnosis of osteoporosis, monitoring of BMD measurement) and in medical research in several situations (e.g. assessment of morphological asymmetry in athletes, estimation of resting energy expenditure, consequences of dietary protein or disabilities of the central nervous system on BMD and body composition, assessment of vertebral strength and vertebral fracture risk, or study of dry bones such as the ulna). It will certainly help the researchers and/or physicians using DXA to improve their knowledge of the wide range of potential uses that this technique allows.

Prof. A. El Maghraoui
Rheumatology Department,
Military Hospital Mohammed V,
Rabat,
Morocco

Part 1

Bone Mineral Density

1

Interpreting a DXA Scan in Clinical Practice

Abdellah El Maghraoui
Rheumatology Department, Military Hospital Mohammed V, Rabat, Morocco

1. Introduction

Osteoporosis is a metabolic bone disorder characterized by low bone mass and microarchitectural deterioration, with a subsequent increase in bone fragility and susceptibility to fracture. Dual-energy x-ray absorptiometry (DXA) is recognized as the reference method to measure bone mineral density (BMD) with acceptable accuracy errors and good precision and reproducibility(Blake and Fogelman 2007). The World Health Organization (WHO) has established DXA as the best densitometric technique for assessing BMD in postmenopausal women and based the definitions of osteopenia and osteoporosis on its results (table 1)(Kanis 1994; Kanis, Borgstrom et al. 2005). DXA allows accurate diagnosis of osteoporosis, estimation of fracture risk, and monitoring of patients undergoing treatment. Additional features of DXA include measurement of BMD at multiple skeletal sites, safety of performance, short investigation time, and ease of use(Hans, Downs et al. 2006; Lewiecki, Binkley et al. 2006). A DXA measurement can be completed in about 5 minutes with minimal radiation exposure (about one tenth that of a standard chest x-ray for a quick hips and spine exam).

Diagnosis	*T-score*
Normal	>-1.0
Osteopenia	<-1.0, >-2.5
Osteoporosis	<-2.5
Severe osteoporosis	<-2.5 plus fragility fractures

Table 1. WHO Osteoporosis Classification

2. Principle of DXA scanning

As with many other diagnostic examinations, DXA scans should be critically assessed by the interpreting physician and densitometrist for abnormalities that may affect BMD measurements. In clinical practice, recognition of diverse artifacts and disease processes that may influence BMD results can be of major importance in the optimal interpretation of DXA scans(Roux 1998). Physicians not directly involved in the performance and interpretation of DXA should be familiar enough to detect common positioning and scanning problems, to know what should appear on a report, what questions to ask if the necessary information is not on the report, how to apply the results in patient management, and when to do and how to interpret a second measurement to monitor treatment(Watts 2004).

Several different types of DXA systems are available, but they all operate on similar principles. A radiation source is aimed at a radiation detector placed directly opposite the site to be measured. The patient is placed on a table in the path of the radiation beam. The source/detector assembly is then scanned across the measurement region. The attenuation of the radiation beam is determined and is related to the BMD (Blake and Fogelman 2002; Blake and Fogelman 2003).

Because DXA scanners use two X-ray energies in the presence of three types of tissue (bone mineral, lean tissue and adipose tissue), there are considerable errors arising from the inhomogeneous distribution of adipose tissue in the human body(Tothill and Avenell 1994) (which can be studied either through cadaver studies(Svendsen, Hassager et al. 1995), CT imaging to delineate the distribution of adipose tissue external to bone(Kuiper, van Kuijk et al. 1996; Lee, Wren et al. 2007) or MRI to measure the percentage of marrow fat inside bone(Griffith, Yeung et al. 2006)). These studies suggest BMD measurement errors of around 5 to 8%.

DXA technology can measure virtually any skeletal site, but clinical use has been concentrated on the lumbar spine, proximal femur, forearm, and total body (Hans, Downs et al. 2006). DXA systems are available as either full table systems (capable of multiple skeletal measurements, including the spine and hip) or as peripheral systems (limited to measuring the peripheral skeleton). Because of their versatility, and the ability to measure the skeletal sites of greatest clinical interest, full table DXA systems are the current clinical choice for osteoporosis assessment. Peripheral DXA systems, portable and less expensive than full table systems, are more frequently used as screening and early risk assessment tools; they cannot be used for treatments follow-up. Spine and proximal femur scans represent the majority of the clinical measurements performed using DXA. Most full table DXA systems are able to perform additional scans, including lateral spine BMD measurements, body composition study, assessment of vertebral fractures, measurements of children and infants, assessment of bone around prosthetic implants, small-animal studies and measurements of excised bone specimens. However, for children measurement, the exam should be undertaken by clinicians skilled in interpretation of scans in children in centers that have an adapted paediatric software.

Early DXA systems used a pencil beam geometry and a single detector, which was scanned across the measurement region. Modern full table DXA scanners use a fan-beam source and multiple detectors, which are swept across the measurement region. Fan beam provides the advantage of decreased scan times compared to single-beam systems, but these machines typically cost more because of the need for multiple X-ray detectors. Fan-beam systems use either a single-view or multiview mode to image the skeleton (Lewiecki and Borges 2006).

In clinical practice, BMD measurements are widely used to diagnose osteoporosis and measurement in bone mass are commonly used as a surrogate for fracture risk (Price, Walters et al. 2003). BMD is the measured parameter, and allows the calculation of the bone mineral content (BMC) in grams and the two-dimensional projected area in cm^2 of the bone(s) being measured; thus the units of BMD are g/cm^2. The BMD values (in g/cm^2) are not used for diagnosing osteoporosis. Instead, a working group of the WHO proposed to define osteoporosis on the basis of the T-score (which is the difference between the measured BMD and the mean value of young adults, expressed in standard deviations (SD) for a normal population of the same gender and ethnicity)(Watts 2004). Despite its limitations; this definition, which concerns only postmenopausal women and men over 50, is currently applied worldwide. Thus, the WHO diagnostic criteria for osteoporosis define osteoporosis in terms of a T-score below −2.5 and osteopenia when T-score is between -2.5 and -1.

The T-score is calculated using the formula: (patient's BMD - young normal mean)/SD of young normal. For example, if a patient has a BMD of 0.700 g/cm^2, the young normal mean is 1.000 g/cm^2, and the young normal standard deviation is 0.100 g/cm^2, then this patient's T-score would be (0.700 - 1.000)/0.100, or –0.300/0.100, or –3.0(Watts 2004). A T-score of 0 is equal to the young normal mean value, -1.0 is 1 SD low, -2.0 is 2 SD low, etc. Although the WHO classification was not intended to be applied to individual patients, it works well to define "normal" (T-score –1.0 and above) and "osteoporosis" (T-score –2.5 and below). Several large studies have shown an unacceptably high risk of fracture in post-menopausal women who have T-scores of –2.5 and below. Thus, this threshold is the cornerstone of the patient's assessment. For the therapeutic decisions, however, other risk factors are considered such as prevalent fractures, age and low body mass index.

In addition to the T-scores, DXA reports also provide Z-scores, which are calculated similarly to the T-score, except that the patient's BMD is compared with an age-matched (and race- and gender-matched) mean, and the result expressed as a standard deviation score(Watts 2004). In premenopausal women, a low Z-score (below -2.0) indicates that bone density is lower than expected and should trigger a search for an underlying cause.

3. Who should have a DXA measurement?

Most official groups recommend screening healthy women for osteoporosis at age 65, and testing higher-risk women earlier(Baddoura, Awada et al. 2006). In Europe the recommendations are to screen for risk factors of osteoporosis and to perform BMD measurement in women with such risks. The International Society for Clinical Densitometry (ISCD) recommends screening men without risk factors for osteoporosis at age 70, and screening higher-risk men earlier. Risk factors include dementia, poor health, recent falls, prolonged immobilization, smoking, alcohol abuse, low body weight, history of fragility fracture in a first-degree relative, estrogen deficiency at an early age (<45 years), and steroid use for more than 3 months. Of course, BMD testing is an appropriate tool in the evaluation of patients who have diseases (e.g. hyperthyroidism, hyperparathyroidism, celiac disease, etc.) or use medications (e.g. glucocorticoids, GnRH agonists, aromatase inhibitors etc.) that might cause bone loss. Another indication is radiographic evidence of "osteopenia" or a vertebral fracture).

Recently, many epidemiological studies have validated risk assessment indices for osteoporosis in women. The purpose of the risk assessment indices is not to diagnose osteoporosis or low BMD, but to identify women who are more likely to have low BMD (Hillier, Stone et al. 2007). Such indices, while not identifying all cases of osteoporosis, increase the efficiency of BMD measurement by focusing on subjects who are at increased risk (Cadarette, Jaglal et al. 2000; Gnudi and Sitta 2005; Salaffi, Silveri et al. 2005). The easiest to use in clinical practice is certainly the Osteoporosis Self-assessment Tool (OST). The calculated risk index is based on self-reported age and weight: [(weight in kilograms – age in years) × 0.2, truncated to an integer]. It was developed and validated in several studies in Asian and White women(Richy, Ethgen et al. 2004; El Maghraoui, Guerboub et al. 2007; El Maghraoui, Habbassi et al. 2007) and men (Adler, Tran et al. 2003; Ghazi, Mounach et al. 2007).

4. Site of measurement of BMD

The ISCD recommends obtaining BMD measurements of the posteroanterior spine and hip(Leib, Binkley et al. 2006). The lateral spine and Ward's triangle region of the hip should not be used for diagnosis, because these sites overestimate osteoporosis and results can be false-positive. Evidence suggests that the femur (neck or total hip) is the optimum site for predicting the risk of hip fracture and the spine is the optimum site for monitoring response to treatment. Thus, many authors recommend hip measure alone for the fracture risk assessment(Kanis, Johnell et al. 2000; Kanis, Oden et al. 2001; Kanis 2002; Johnell, Kanis et al. 2005; Kanis, Seeman et al. 2005; Arabi, Baddoura et al. 2007). In very obese patients, those with primary hyperparathyroidism, or those in whom the hip or the spine, or both, cannot be measured or interpreted, BMD may be measured in the forearm, using a 33% radius on the nondominant forearm.

5. Interpreting a DXA scan

The most important informations to check are the correct identification of the patient, his date of birth and also the sex and ethnicity which are mandatory to calculate T-scores. Sex is used by all manufacturers to calculate T-scores (i.e. T-scores for women are calculated using a female normative database, while T-scores for men are calculated using a male normative database). Although all manufacturers use race in calculating Z-scores, there is inconsistency in the way race is handled when calculating T-scores. Norland and Hologic are using race in calculating T-scores (i.e. T-scores for Caucasians are calculated using a Caucasian normative database, T-scores for Blacks are calculated using a normative database for Blacks); however, GE Lunar and recent Hologic machines use the database for young-normal Caucasians to calculate T-scores, regardless of the race of the subject. The ISCD recommends the latter approach for use in North America (Baim, Wilson et al. 2005) because using race-adjusted T-scores results in a similar prevalence of "osteoporosis" in every racial group, despite the fact that age-specific fracture rates can be very different.

5.1 Positioning

The main purpose of the DXA scan image is to check if the patient is positioned correctly, something that the technologist must determine before the patient leaves the testing centre. Positioning should also be doublechecked by the clinician who interprets the test(Roux 1998). There is many available resources for BMD technologists and physicians training, such as ISCD or International Osteoporosis Foundation (IOF) courses.

A scan with correct positioning of the spine is shown in Fig. 1a: the patient is straight on the table (spine is straight on the image), not rotated (spinous processes are centered), and centered in the field (roughly equal soft tissue fields on either side of the spine). Patients with scoliosis cannot be positioned with the spine straight on the table; moreover with severe scoliosis degenerative changes can occur that invalidate the spine measurement. The scan should extend up sufficiently far to include part of the lowest vertebra with ribs (which is usually T12) and low enough to show the pelvic brim (which is usually the level of the L4–L5 interspace). Most testing centers will elevate the patient's knees with a foam block (hip at a 90° angle to the spine) to try to partially flatten the normal lumbar lordosis. For proper positioning of the hip, the patient should have the femur straight on the table (shaft parallel to the edge of the picture), with 15–25° of internal rotation, which can be achieved by the use of positioning devices. Internal rotation may be improved by having the patient flex the foot before doing the internal rotation, and then relaxing the foot after the strap is in place. This amount of internal rotation presents the long axis of the femoral neck perpendicular to the X-ray beam, providing the greatest area and the lowest bone mineral content (and the lowest BMD), and is confirmed on the scan by seeing little or none of the lesser trochanter (Fig. 1b)(Lekamwasam and Lenora 2003; 2004). If the desired amount of internal rotation cannot be achieved, as is often the case in patients with hip arthritis or short femoral necks, the technologist should place the patient comfortably in a position that is likely to be reproducible in a subsequent scan (Hamdy, Kiebzak et al. 2006; Lewiecki, Binkley et al. 2006).

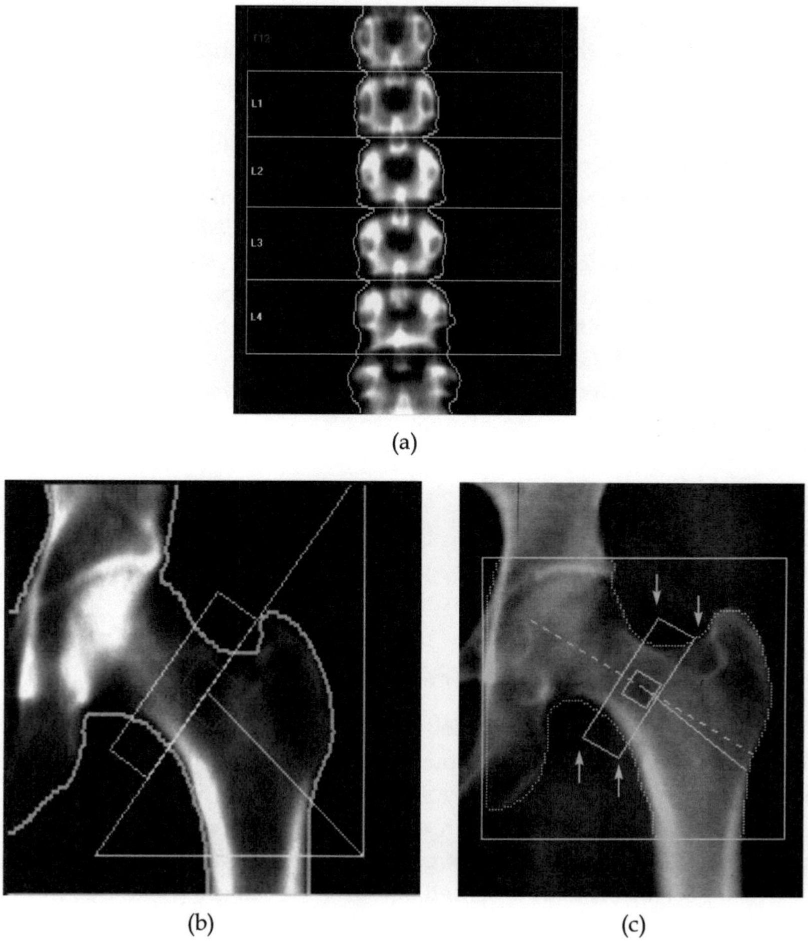

Fig. 1. Correct positioning and analysis of the L1–L4 spine (a) and the proximal femur (Lunar (b) and Hologic (c)).

5.2 DXA scan analysis

The software marks regions of interest in the spine and hip, but the technologist can and should make adjustments if needed. The spine region of interest consists of the L1 through L4 vertebrae (Fig. 1a). Correct placement of the top and bottom of the spine ''box'' is critical.

The intervertebral lines can be moved or angled, if necessary. There must be sufficient soft tissue on both sides of the spine; otherwise BMD will be under estimated. The hip regions of interest include the femoral neck, trochanter, and total hip (Fig. 1b). Ward's region and the intertrochanteric region are not relevant (and can be deleted from the results reports. The default hip analysis includes a midline that must be placed correctly for the other sites to be identified correctly. The preferred position for the rectangular femoral neck box differs for the different manufacturers. For GE Lunar, the femoral neck box is located by the analysis program at the narrowest and lowest density section of the neck; typically this will be about half way between the femoral head and the trochanter (Fig. 1b). For Hologic the box is on the distal part of the femoral neck (Fig. 1c). This induces a large difference among these 2 measurements, because of a gradient of BMD all along the femoral neck (the proximal being the highest, the distal being the lowest). Thus careful checking of the femoral neck box is mandatory.

The image should be evaluated for artifacts (e.g. surgical clips, navel rings, barium sulphate, metal from zipper, coin, clip, or other metallic object) or local structural change (e.g. osteophytes, syndesmophytes, compression fractures, aortic calcification). Almost all artifacts and local structural change will spuriously elevate BMD(El Maghraoui 2004). This is especially true for spinal degenerative change, which can elevate spine BMD by 2, 3, or more T-score. In the spine, absent bone (laminectomy or spina bifida) or vertebral rotation (idiopathic scoliosis) will spuriously lower BMD. All evaluable vertebrae should be used, but vertebrae that are affected by local structural change should be deleted from the analysis. Most agree that decisions can be based on two vertebrae; the use of a single vertebra is not recommended. If all vertebrae are affected, the spine should be reported as "invalid," with no BMD or T-score results given. Figure 2 and 3 show examples from common spine and hips scanning problems.

Finally, physicians must keep in mind to actively look for secondary osteoporosis in front of low BMD value, either by thorough history taking or with biochemical studies before stating about post menopausal osteoporosis.

6. Vertebral fracture assessment (VFA)

For assessing vertebral heights (also called vertebral morphometry), a special software is used to determine vertebral body dimensions. The computer (with the help of the technologist) places points on the superior and inferior endplates of each vertebra. The vertebral heights are calculated and compared to each other as well as to the expected normal dimensions. With the advent of higher-resolution DXA systems, visual assessment of fractures is also possible from DXA-based lateral spine images (Figure 4). In this situation, the DXA system essentially functions as a digital X-ray imaging device. Visual assessment is performed from a computer monitor or high-resolution printout. To optimize the assessment, the use of high-definition dual-energy images has been recommended (Rea, Li et al. 2000; Chapurlat, Duboeuf et al. 2006; Olenginski, Newman et al. 2006). Using a DXA system for assessing vertebral fracture status has several advantages. The evaluation of spine fractures can be performed without a conventional lateral spine X-ray. This can be done at the same time and at the same place as the BMD measurement, with much less radiation than a conventional spine X-ray. Moreover, VFA is a technology for diagnosing vertebral fractures that may alter diagnostic classification, improve fracture risk stratification,

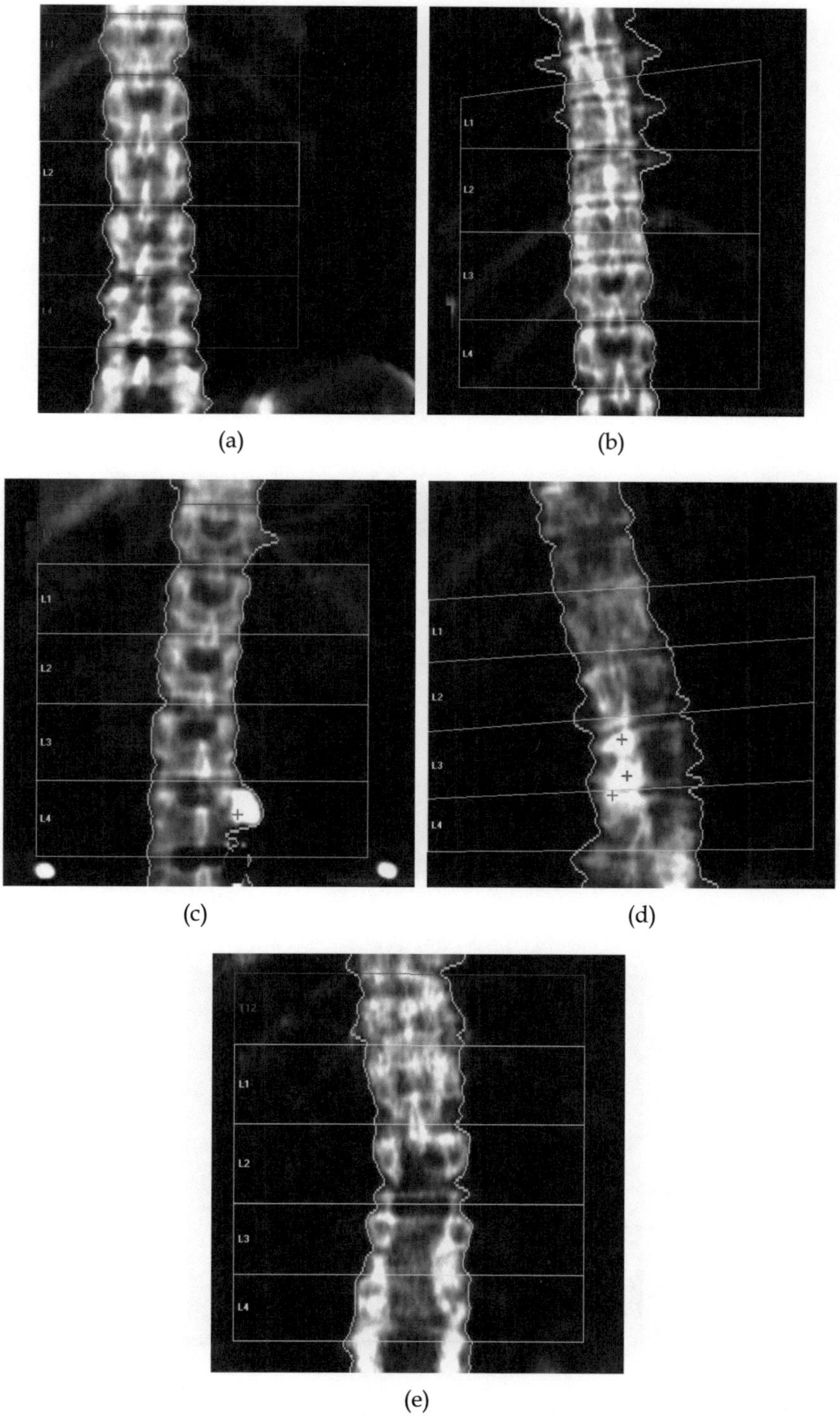

Fig. 2. Examples among some common spine scanning problems: (a) The spine is too close to the right side of the image (b) Vertebral levels are mis-identified (c) Metal button over L4 (d) Scoliosis, and osteophyte at L3–L4 (e) Laminectomy

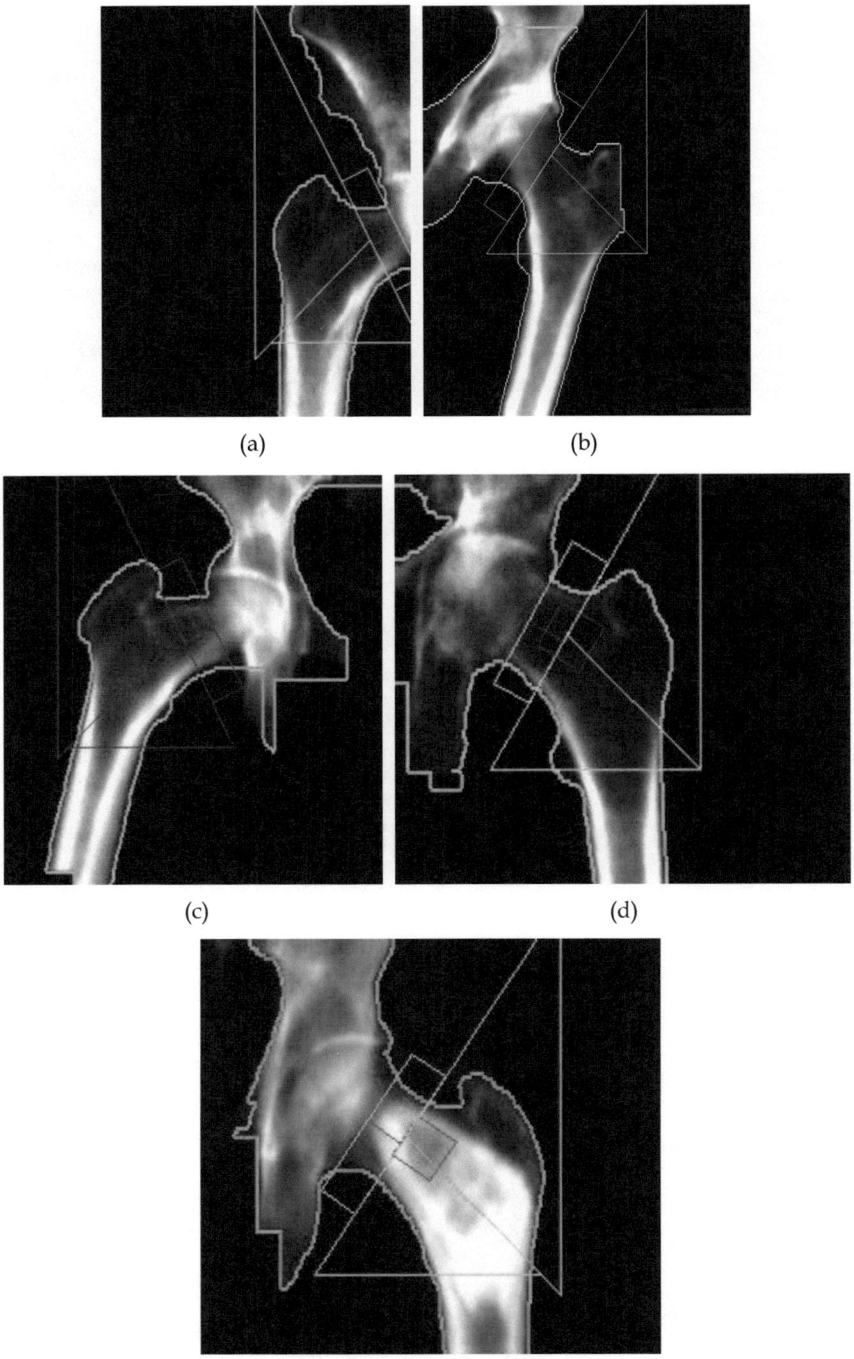

(a) (b)

(c) (d)

(e)

Fig. 3. Examples among some common hip scanning problems: (a) The scan did not go far enough laterally and part of the femoral head is missing. (b) The femur is adducted (c) The femur is abducted (d) Suboptimal internal rotation (too much of the lesser trochanter is showing) (e) Abnormal bone (history of hip fracture and osteosynthesis)

and identify patients likely to benefit from pharmacological therapy who otherwise might not be treated(Olenginski, Newman et al. 2006; Roux, Fechtenbaum et al. 2007). Despite the apparent advantages, the future of VFA using DXA remains unclear. Skeletal radiologists have criticized the technique for being insensitive and inaccurate for detecting vertebral fractures in particular at the upper thoracic spine. A DXA image is of lower resolution than a conventional X-ray and might fail to identify other potential problems or diseases that would be apparent on a spine film. However, VFA allows ruling out vertebral fracture at levels where vertebral fracture is most common, i.e. the lumbar and the mid and lower thoracic levels, and the pencil beam mode of assessment eliminates parallax errors in viewing the vertebral body, which can sometimes make a normal vertebral body appear to have been compressed in a routine spine x-ray(Duboeuf, Bauer et al. 2005; Jacobs-Kosmin, Sandorfi et al. 2005; Chapurlat, Duboeuf et al. 2006; Damiano, Kolta et al. 2006).

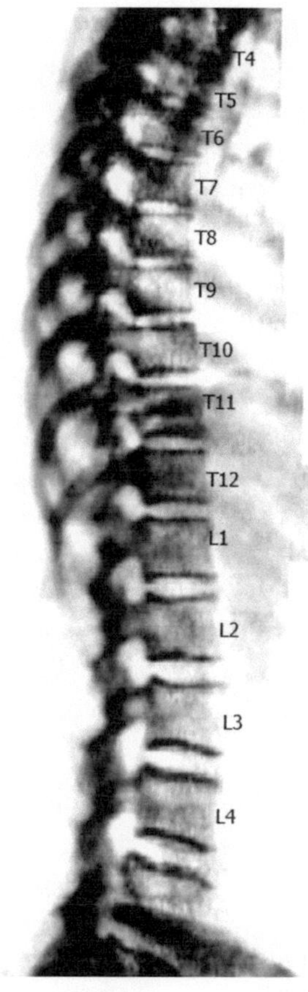

Fig. 4. Vertebral fracture assessment from a dual x-ray absorptiometry image of the spine.

At this time, DXA devices are not generally accepted as a surrogate for spinal X-rays, though they may provide a useful screening tool in higher-risk patients when spinal X-rays are unavailable. For example, individuals over 65, subjects reporting significant height loss or patients on long term glucocorticoid therapy who have not had previous vertebral fractures or spinal radiographs could benefit from a VFA.

7. Concordance between measurement sites

It is recommended to measure the PA lumbar spine and proximal femur and classifying the patient based on the lowest T-score from three sites (lumbar spine, femoral neck, and total hip). Although the BMDs at different anatomic regions are correlated, the agreement between sites is low when it comes to classifying individual subjects as osteoporotic or not. Thus, T-score discordance between the lumbar spine and hip testing sites is a commonly observed phenomenon in densitometery. T-score discordance is the observation that the T-score of an individual patient varies from one key measurement site to another.

7.1 Prevalence and risk factors of T-score discordance

Various studies have analyzed the prevalence and impact of T-score discordance on the management of osteoporosis(Faulkner, von Stetten et al. 1999; Woodson 2000; O'Gradaigh, Debiram et al. 2003; Moayyeri, Soltani et al. 2005). Only two studies focused on risk factors of this commonly observed discordance (Moayyeri, Soltani et al. 2005; El Maghraoui, Mouinga Abayi et al. 2007; El Maghraoui, Mouinga Abayi et al. 2007). Five different causes for occurrence of discordance between the spine and the hip sites have been described(Woodson 2000).

1. Physiologic discordance is related to the skeleton's natural adaptive reaction to normal external and internal factors and forces. Mechanical strain especially related to weight bearing plays a key role in this kind of discordance. An example of this type of discordance is the difference observed between the dominant and non-dominant total hip(Hamdy, Kiebzak et al. 2006). The explanation is that weight bearing can cause rise in bone density especially in the hip and femur regions. Moreover, the spine and hips usually start out with different T-scores (the spine is said to reach peak at least 5 yrs before the hip)(Blank, Malone et al. 2006). And finally, bone loss observed with age in an individual may be more rapid and important in trabecular than cortical bone is another explanation(Agarwal and Camacho 2006). Trabecular bones (typical of lumbar area) are known to have a more rapid rate of deprivation in early post-menopausal state in comparison to cortical bone (typical of proximal femur).
2. The second type of discordance described as pathophysiologic discordance is seen secondary to a disease. Common examples observed in the elderly include vertebral osteophytosis, vertebral end plate and facet sclerosis, osteochondrosis, and aortic calcification(Bolotin 2001; Theodorou and Theodorou 2002). Another important cause in younger patients is ankylosing spondylitis syndesmophytes(El Maghraoui, Borderie et al. 1999; Maillefert, Aho et al. 2001; El Maghraoui 2004; El Maghraoui 2004; El Maghraoui, Do Santos Zounon et al. 2005). The abnormal calcium deposition within the field of the DXA region of interest (ROI) leads to the falsely elevated spine T-score. A second subtype is a true discordance resulting from a more decreased BMD in the lumbar spine than the hips. Indeed, most of the aetiologies of the secondary osteoporosis (such as glucocorticoid excess, hyperthyroidism, malabsorption, liver disease, rheumatoid arthritis) first affect spinal column(El

Maghraoui 2004; Khan, Hanley et al. 2006). This will lead to higher prevalence of lumbar osteoporosis.

3. Anatomic discordance is owing to differences in the composition of bone envelopes tested. An example is the difference in T-scores found for the posteroanterior lumbar spine and the supine lateral lumbar spine in the same patient.
4. Artifactual discordance occurs when dense synthetic manmade substances are within the field of ROI of the test: e.g. barium sulphate, metal from zipper, coin, clip, or other metallic object.
5. And finally, technical discordance occurs because of device errors, technician variability, patients' movements, and variation due to other unpredictable sources. With respect to positioning error, some studies showed that either excessive internal or external rotation of the femur during test acquisition resulted in a BMD difference of as much as 10% compared with correct positioning. We demonstrated in a previous study that DXA in vivo reproducibility is two-fold better in the hips than the spine especially when measuring both hips(El Maghraoui, Do Santos Zounon et al. 2005). Finally, technical discordance can occur due to the normative reference data used by the device software to analyze the test(Liao, Wu et al. 2003; McMahon, Nightingale et al. 2004; Lewiecki, Binkley et al. 2006). This type of discordance occurs when the average BMD of the normative group used to calculate the T-score is significantly different from the average value found for the whole population.

7.2 Consequences of T-score discordance on osteoporosis management

The high prevalence of T-score discordance could induce some problems for the physicians in decision-making regarding these patients. In general, high prevalence of discordance between lumbar spine and hip T-scores suggests some defects in the cut-off values for definition of osteoporosis and osteopenia proposed with the WHO. The inconsistencies in the diagnostic classification of osteoporosis between skeletal sites lend credence to the notion that BMD should be used as only one of the factors in making therapeutic decisions when evaluating patients with osteoporosis. An international team convened by the WHO is trying to develop a globally applicable measure of absolute fracture risk based upon multiple risk factors including BMD. This could silence much of the controversy regarding the choice of reference data for T-score calculation and usefulness of relatively arbitrary densitometric categorizations. However, one can speculate that discordance in individual fracture risk estimation with this new absolute fracture risk will still be observed as it will be based on different sites BMD.

8. Conclusion

Correct performance of BMD measurements using DXA requires rigorous attention to detail in positioning and analysis. When DXA studies are performed incorrectly, it can lead to major mistakes in diagnosis and therapy. Measurement error must be considered when evaluating serial assessments. A clear understanding of the interpretation of serial measurements and the statistical principles impacting upon their interpretation is necessary to determine whether a change is real and not simply random fluctuation. Moreover, it is important to keep in mind that fracture-protection benefit may be realized before BMD gains are detected. Physicians interested in osteoporosis management, even if not directly involved in the performance and interpretation of DXA, should be familiar with the principles outlined here to minimize serious errors and allow proper use of bone densitometry.

9. Abbreviations

BMC: bone mineral content

BMD: bone mineral density

CV: coefficient of variation

DXA: dual-energy x-ray absorptiometry

IOF: international osteoporosis foundation

ISCD: international society for clinical densitometry

LSC: least significant change

OST: osteoporosis self-assessment tool

PE: precision error

ROI: region of interest

SD: standard deviation

SDD: smallest detectable difference

VFA: vertebral fracture assessment

WHO: world health organization

10. References

Adler, R. A., M. T. Tran, et al. (2003). "Performance of the Osteoporosis Self-assessment Screening Tool for osteoporosis in American men." *Mayo Clin Proc* 78(6): 723-7.

Agarwal, M. and P. Camacho (2006). "Bone densitometry. Interpretation and pitfalls." *Postgrad Med* 119(1): 17-23.

Arabi, A., R. Baddoura, et al. (2007). "Discriminative ability of dual-energy X-ray absorptiometry site selection in identifying patients with osteoporotic fractures." *Bone* 40(4): 1060-5.

Baddoura, R., H. Awada, et al. (2006). "An audit of bone densitometry practice with reference to ISCD, IOF and NOF guidelines." *Osteoporos Int* 17(7): 1111-5.

Baim, S., C. R. Wilson, et al. (2005). "Precision assessment and radiation safety for dual-energy X-ray absorptiometry: position paper of the International Society for Clinical Densitometry." *J Clin Densitom* 8(4): 371-8.

Blake, G. M. and I. Fogelman (2002). "Dual energy x-ray absorptiometry and its clinical applications." *Semin Musculoskelet Radiol* 6(3): 207-18.

Blake, G. M. and I. Fogelman (2003). "DXA scanning and its interpretation in osteoporosis." *Hosp Med* 64(9): 521-5.

Blake, G. M. and I. Fogelman (2007). "The role of DXA bone density scans in the diagnosis and treatment of osteoporosis." *Postgrad Med J* 83(982): 509-517.

Blank, R. D., D. G. Malone, et al. (2006). "Patient variables impact lumbar spine dual energy X-ray absorptiometry precision." *Osteoporos Int* 17(5): 768-74.

Bolotin, H. H. (2001). "Inaccuracies inherent in dual-energy X-ray absorptiometry in vivo bone mineral densitometry may flaw osteopenic/osteoporotic interpretations and mislead assessment of antiresorptive therapy effectiveness." *Bone* 28(5): 548-55.

Cadarette, S. M., S. B. Jaglal, et al. (2000). "Development and validation of the Osteoporosis Risk Assessment Instrument to facilitate selection of women for bone densitometry." *Cmaj* 162(9): 1289-94.

Chapurlat, R. D., F. Duboeuf, et al. (2006). "Effectiveness of instant vertebral assessment to detect prevalent vertebral fracture." *Osteoporos Int* 17(8): 1189-95.

Damiano, J., S. Kolta, et al. (2006). "Diagnosis of vertebral fractures by vertebral fracture assessment." *J Clin Densitom* 9(1): 66-71.

Duboeuf, F., D. C. Bauer, et al. (2005). "Assessment of vertebral fracture using densitometric morphometry." *J Clin Densitom* 8(3): 362-8.

El Maghraoui, A. (2004). "L'ostéoprose cortisonique." *Presse Med* 33(17): 1213-7.

El Maghraoui, A. (2004). "La spondylarthrite ankylosante." *Presse Med* 33(20): 1459-64.

El Maghraoui, A. (2004). "Osteoporosis and ankylosing spondylitis." *Joint Bone Spine* 71(4): 291-5.

El Maghraoui, A., D. Borderie, et al. (1999). "Osteoporosis, body composition, and bone turnover in ankylosing spondylitis." *J Rheumatol* 26(10): 2205-9.

El Maghraoui, A., A. A. Do Santos Zounon, et al. (2005). "Reproducibility of bone mineral density measurements using dual X-ray absorptiometry in daily clinical practice." *Osteoporos Int* 16(12): 1742-8.

El Maghraoui, A., A. A. Guerboub, et al. (2007). "Body mass index and gynecological factors as determinants of bone mass in healthy Moroccan women." *Maturitas* 56(4): 375-82.

El Maghraoui, A., A. Habbassi, et al. (2007). "Validation and comparative evaluation of four osteoporosis risk indexes in Moroccan menopausal women." *Arch Osteop* (in press).

El Maghraoui, A., D. A. Mouinga Abayi, et al. (2007). "Prevalence and risk factors of discordance in diagnosis of osteoporosis using spine and hip bone densitometry." *Ann Rheum Dis* 66: 271-2.

El Maghraoui, A., D. A. Mouinga Abayi, et al. (2007). "Discordance in diagnosis of osteoporosis using spine and hip bone densitometry." *J Clin Densitom* (in press).

Faulkner, K. G., E. von Stetten, et al. (1999). "Discordance in patient classification using T-scores." *J Clin Densitom* 2(3): 343-50.

Ghazi, M., A. Mounach, et al. (2007). "Performance of the osteoporosis risk assessment tool in Moroccan men." *Clin Rheumatol.*

Gnudi, S. and E. Sitta (2005). "Clinical risk factor evaluation to defer postmenopausal women from bone mineral density measurement: an Italian study." *J Clin Densitom* 8(2): 199-205.

Griffith, J. F., D. K. Yeung, et al. (2006). "Vertebral marrow fat content and diffusion and perfusion indexes in women with varying bone density: MR evaluation." *Radiology* 241(3): 831-8.

Hamdy, R., G. M. Kiebzak, et al. (2006). "The prevalence of significant left-right differences in hip bone mineral density." *Osteoporos Int* 17(12): 1772-80.

Hans, D., R. W. Downs, Jr., et al. (2006). "Skeletal sites for osteoporosis diagnosis: the 2005 ISCD Official Positions." *J Clin Densitom* 9(1): 15-21.

Hillier, T. A., K. L. Stone, et al. (2007). "Evaluating the value of repeat bone mineral density measurement and prediction of fractures in older women: the study of osteoporotic fractures." *Arch Intern Med* 167(2): 155-60.

Jacobs-Kosmin, D., N. Sandorfi, et al. (2005). "Vertebral deformities identified by vertebral fracture assessment: associations with clinical characteristics and bone mineral density." *J Clin Densitom* 8(3): 267-72.

Johnell, O., J. A. Kanis, et al. (2005). "Predictive value of BMD for hip and other fractures." *J Bone Miner Res* 20(7): 1185-94.

Kanis, J. A. (1994). "Assessment of fracture risk and its application to screening for postmenopausal osteoporosis: synopsis of a WHO report. WHO Study Group." *Osteoporos Int* 4(6): 368-81.

Kanis, J. A. (2002). "Diagnosis of osteoporosis and assessment of fracture risk." *Lancet* 359(9321): 1929-36.

Kanis, J. A., F. Borgstrom, et al. (2005). "Assessment of fracture risk." *Osteoporos Int* 16(6): 581-9.

Kanis, J. A., O. Johnell, et al. (2000). "Risk of hip fracture according to the World Health Organization criteria for osteopenia and osteoporosis." *Bone* 27(5): 585-90.

Kanis, J. A., A. Oden, et al. (2001). "The burden of osteoporotic fractures: a method for setting intervention thresholds." *Osteoporos Int* 12(5): 417-27.

Kanis, J. A., E. Seeman, et al. (2005). "The perspective of the International Osteoporosis Foundation on the official positions of the International Society for Clinical Densitometry." *Osteoporos Int* 16(5): 456-9, discussion 579-80.

Khan, A. A., D. A. Hanley, et al. (2006). "Standards for performing DXA in individuals with secondary causes of osteoporosis." *J Clin Densitom* 9(1): 47-57.

Kuiper, J. W., C. van Kuijk, et al. (1996). "Accuracy and the influence of marrow fat on quantitative CT and dual-energy X-ray absorptiometry measurements of the femoral neck in vitro." *Osteoporos Int* 6(1): 25-30.

Lee, D. C., T. A. L. Wren, et al. (2007). "Correcting DXA pediatric bone mineral density measurments to account for fat inhomogeneity." *ASBMR* W514: (Abstract).

Leib, E. S., N. Binkley, et al. (2006). "Position Development Conference of the International Society for Clinical Densitometry. Vancouver, BC, July 15-17, 2005." *J Rheumatol* 33(11): 2319-21.

Lekamwasam, S. and R. S. Lenora (2003). "Effect of leg rotation on hip bone mineral density measurements." *J Clin Densitom* 6(4): 331-6.

Lewiecki, E. M., N. Binkley, et al. (2006). "DXA quality matters." *J Clin Densitom* 9(4): 388-92.

Lewiecki, E. M. and J. L. Borges (2006). "Bone density testing in clinical practice." *Arq Bras Endocrinol Metabol* 50(4): 586-95.

Liao, E. Y., X. P. Wu, et al. (2003). "Establishment and evaluation of bone mineral density reference databases appropriate for diagnosis and evaluation of osteoporosis in Chinese women." *J Bone Miner Metab* 21(3): 184-92.

Maillefert, J. F., L. S. Aho, et al. (2001). "Changes in bone density in patients with ankylosing spondylitis: a two-year follow-up study." *Osteoporos Int* 12(7): 605-9.

McMahon, K., J. Nightingale, et al. (2004). "Discordance in DXA male reference ranges." *J Clin Densitom* 7(2): 121-6.

Moayyeri, A., A. Soltani, et al. (2005). "Discordance in diagnosis of osteoporosis using spine and hip bone densitometry." *BMC Endocr Disord* 5(1): 3.

O'Gradaigh, D., I. Debiram, et al. (2003). "A prospective study of discordance in diagnosis of osteoporosis using spine and proximal femur bone densitometry." *Osteoporos Int* 14(1): 13-8.

Olenginski, T. P., E. D. Newman, et al. (2006). "Development and evaluation of a vertebral fracture assessment program using IVA and its integration with mobile DXA." *J Clin Densitom* 9(1): 72-7.

Price, R. I., M. J. Walters, et al. (2003). "Impact of the analysis of a bone density reference range on determination of the T-score." *J Clin Densitom* 6(1): 51-62.

Rea, J. A., J. Li, et al. (2000). "Visual assessment of vertebral deformity by X-ray absorptiometry: a highly predictive method to exclude vertebral deformity." *Osteoporos Int* 11(8): 660-8.

Richy, F., O. Ethgen, et al. (2004). "Primary prevention of osteoporosis: mass screening scenario or prescreening with questionnaires? An economic perspective." *J Bone Miner Res* 19(12): 1955-60.

Roux, C. (1998). "Densitométrie osseuse et ostéoporose." *J Radiol* 79(9): 821-3.

Roux, C., J. Fechtenbaum, et al. (2007). "Mild prevalent and incident vertebral fractures are risk factors for new fractures." *Osteoporos Int.*

Salaffi, F., F. Silveri, et al. (2005). "Development and validation of the osteoporosis prescreening risk assessment (OPERA) tool to facilitate identification of women likely to have low bone density." *Clin Rheumatol* 24(3): 203-11.

Svendsen, O. L., C. Hassager, et al. (1995). "Impact of soft tissue on in vivo accuracy of bone mineral measurements in the spine, hip, and forearm: a human cadaver study." *J Bone Miner Res* 10(6): 868-73.

Theodorou, D. J. and S. J. Theodorou (2002). "Dual-energy X-ray absorptiometry in clinical practice: application and interpretation of scans beyond the numbers." *Clin Imaging* 26(1): 43-9.

Tothill, P. and A. Avenell (1994). "Errors in dual-energy X-ray absorptiometry of the lumbar spine owing to fat distribution and soft tissue thickness during weight change." *Br J Radiol* 67(793): 71-5.

Watts, N. B. (2004). "Fundamentals and pitfalls of bone densitometry using dual-energy X-ray absorptiometry (DXA)." *Osteoporos Int* 15(11): 847-54.

Woodson, G. (2000). "Dual X-ray absorptiometry T-score concordance and discordance between the hip and spine measurement sites." *J Clin Densitom* 3(4): 319-24.

2

Monitoring DXA Measurement in Clinical Practice

Abdellah El Maghraoui
Rheumatology Department, Military Hospital Mohammed V, Rabat, Morocco

1. Introduction

Osteoporosis is a worldwide major public health problem. Bone densitometry has become the "gold standard" in its diagnosis and treatment evaluation(El Maghraoui and Roux 2008). With its advantages of high precision, short scan times, low radiation dose, and stable calibration, dual-energy x-ray absorptiometry (DXA) has been established by the World Health Organization (WHO) as the technique of reference for assessing bone mineral density (BMD) in postmenopausal women and based the definitions of osteopenia and osteoporosis on its results. Recently, efficient therapeutic options for treatment of osteoporosis have been developed which create possibilities of effective intervention. Therefore, screening for and treatment of osteoporosis are widely practised in postmenopausal women and in people with an increased risk of osteoporosis because of underlying diseases (e.g. chronic rheumatic diseases especially when treated by corticosteroids)(Phillipov, Seaborn et al. 2001). Moreover, BMD measurement is needed to select patients for osteoporosis treatment, as there is no proof that drugs for osteoporosis (other than hormone replacement therapy [HRT]) are beneficial in women with clinical risk factors for fractures but normal BMD values.

It has also become more and more common to perform a second DXA measurement to monitor BMD status or the effect of therapeutic intervention. When a second measurement is performed on a patient, the clinician needs to distinguish between a true change in BMD and a random fluctuation related to variability in the measurement procedure. The reproducibility of DXA measurements is claimed to be good. Such variability is due to multiple causes, such as device errors, technician variability, patients' movements, and variation due to other unpredictable sources (Nguyen, Sambrook et al. 1997; Lodder, Lems et al. 2004).

The precision error is usually expressed as the coefficient of variation (CV), which is the ratio of the standard deviation (SD) to the mean of the measurements, although several other statistics to express reproducibility exist such as the smallest detectable difference (SDD) or the least significant change (LSC). The SDD represents a cut-off that can be measured in an individual and is usually considered more useful than the CV in clinical practice (Fuleihan, Testa et al. 1995; Ravaud, Reny et al. 1999).

2. Methods of bone mineral density reproducibility measurement

Precision errors are evaluated by performing repeated scans on a representative set of individuals to characterize the reproducibility of the technique. Most published studies examine the short-term precision error, based on repeated measurements of each subject performed over a time period of no more than 2 weeks. Over such a short period, no true change in BMD is expected.

2.1 The coefficient of variation (CV)

The CV, the most commonly presented measure for BMD variability, is the SD corrected for the mean of paired measurements. CV, expressed as a percentage, is calculated as CV (%) = $(\sqrt{((\sum(a-b)^2)/2n)})/((Ma+Mb)/2)x100$ where a and b are the first and the second measurement, Ma and Mb are the mean values for the two groups, and n is the number of paired observations.

Reproducibility is far better for BMD measurement than for most laboratory tests. Reproducibility expressed by the CV is usually 1-2% at the spine on anteroposterior images and 2-3% at the proximal femur in individuals with normal BMD values; the difference between the two sites is ascribable to greater difficulties with repositioning and examining the femur, as compared to the spine. However, these data obtained under nearly experimental conditions may not apply to everyday clinical practice. Reproducibility depends heavily on quality assurance factors, including tests to control the quality and performance of the machine, as well as the experience of the operator. Assessment of machine performance requires daily scanning of a phantom (which may be anthropomorphic or not), followed by calculation of the in vitro coefficient of variation (CV), which serves to evaluate short-term and longterm performance and to detect drift in measurement accuracy. These in vitro data, however, do not necessarily reflect in vivo reproducibility, which should be evaluated at each measurement centre. Measurements are obtained either three times in each of 15 patients or twice in each of 30 patients, and the CV (m/*r*) is calculated from the mean (m) and standard deviation *(r)* of these repeated measurements. The CV is expressed as a percentage and depends on mean BMD values(Phillipov, Seaborn et al. 2001). The standard deviation reflects measurement error, which is a characteristic of machine performance and is independent from the value measured.

2.2 The least significant change (LSC)

For two point measurements in time, a BMD change exceeding $2\sqrt{2}$ times the precision error (PE) of a technique is considered a significant change (with 95% confidence): the corresponding change criterion has been termed "least significant change" or LSC. LSC = 2.8 x PE; where PE is the largest precision error of the technique used (or more easily the CV expressed in percentage). This smallest change that is considered statistically significant is also expressed in percentage(Gluer 1999).

2.3 The smallest detectable difference (SDD)

The measurement error can be calculated using Bland and Altman's 95% limits of agreement method(Bland and Altman 1986). Precision expressed by this method gives an absolute and metric estimate of random measurement error, also called SDD. In this case, where there are two observations for each subject, the standard deviation of the differences (SD_{diff}) estimates the within variability of the measurements. Most disagreements between measurements are expected to be between limits called "limits of agreement" defined as $d \pm z_{(1-a/2)}\ SD_{diff}$ where d is the mean difference between the pairs of measurements and $z_{(1-a/2)}$ is the 100(1-a/2)th centile of the normal distribution. The value d is an estimate of the mean systematic bias of measurement 1 to measurement 2. d is expected to be 0 because a true change in BMD is not assumed to occur during the interval between the two BMD measurements. Defining a to be 5%, the limits of agreement are $+1.96SD_{diff}$ and $-1.96SD_{diff}$. Thus, about twice the standard deviation (SD) of the difference scores gives the 95% limits of agreement for the two measurements by the machine. A test is considered to be capable of detecting a difference, in absolute units, of at least the magnitude of the limits of agreement.

3. Clinical implications of bone mineral density reproducibility measurement

In clinical practice, two absolute values (g/cm^2) have to be compared, rather than two percentages (T-scores). When serial measurements are obtained in a patient, only changes greater than the LSC (in %) or the SDD (in g/cm^2) can be ascribed to treatment effects. Smaller changes may be related to measurement error.

We studied recently the in vivo short term variability of BMD measurement by DXA in three groups of subjects with a wide range of BMD values: healthy young volunteers, postmenopausal women and patients with chronic rheumatic diseases (most of them taking corticosteroids). In all studied subjects, reproducibility expressed by different means was good and independent from clinical and BMD status. Thus, the clinician interpreting a repeated DXA scan of a subject should be aware that a BMD change exceeding the LSC is significant, in our centre arising from a BMD change of at least 3.56% at the total hip and 5.60% at the spine. Expressed as SDD, a BMD change should exceed 0.02 g/cm^2 at the total hip and 0.04 g/cm^2 at the spine before it can be considered a significant change(El Maghraoui, Do Santos Zounon et al. 2005). Indeed, it has become usual to perform repeated DXA measurement: in postmenopausal women to monitor efficacy of treatment and in patients with chronic rheumatic diseases where high prevalence of bone loss has been demonstrated (Maillefert, Aho et al. 2001; Johnson, Petkov et al. 2005) especially when long term corticosteroid therapy is used. In the reports published, variability is usually expressed as CV and the figures for short term variability are lower than the ones we found [7-9]. However, two studies showed variability data more in line with our results. In Ravaud et al.(Ravaud, Reny et al. 1999) study, two samples of healthy (n=70) and elderly (n=57) postmenopausal women showed a CV (%) of 0.9 and 1.8, respectively, at the spine, and of 0.9 and 2.3, respectively, at the total hip. Eastell showed an LSC (%) of 5.4 at the lumbar spine and 8 at the total hip, respectively, in osteoporotic postmenopausal women (Eastell 1996). It has been suggested that the varying results of reproducibility studies might be explained by the "population" investigated; a phantom and healthy young subjects are likely to show more favourable variability than postmenopausal women, possibly in part because of easier positioning for measurement(Gluer, Blake et al. 1995). However, our study failed to show better variability, expressed as CV (%), in young healthy volunteers (El Maghraoui, Do Santos Zounon et al. 2005). Another reason advocated was that osteoarthritis in postmenopausal women may contribute to poorer variability than found in healthy young subjects. The SDD values found in our study were comparable to the figures presented by Ravaud et al. (Ravaud, Reny et al. 1999). In the first group of postmenopausal women (mean age 53 years) they describe, the SDD was 0.02 (g/cm^2) at the total hip and 0.02 at the lumbar spine. In the second group described, women with a mean age of 80 years, these figures were 0.04 and 0.04, respectively. In Lodder et al.(Lodder, Lems et al. 2004) study (Ninety five women, mean age 59.9 years), the SDD was 0.04 (g/cm2) at the total hip and 0.05 at the lumbar spine. The SDD values of the children studied in this study tended to be lower than the values in the postmenopausal women (table I). Using the SDD, one can state that a (BMD) change larger than the figure found is a true (BMD) change in 95% of the cases. The characteristics of the Bland and Altman method thus allow direct insight into the variability of the measurement under study (figure 1).

It has been shown that reproducibility expressed using the SDD is independent of the BMD value whereas reproducibility expressed using the CV or the derived LSC depend on the BMD value. Ravaud et al.(Ravaud, Reny et al. 1999) reported that using SD, the values of the cut-offs are 0.024, 0.030, 0.020, and 0.021 g/cm^2 for postmenopausal women aged ≤70 years and 0.040, 0.033, 0.033, and 0.038 g/cm^2 for postmenopausal osteoporotic women aged >70 years at the spine, femoral neck, greater trochanter, and total hip, respectively. Using CV, cut-offs vary depending on the BMD level. In postmenopausal women aged >70 years, for a BMD level between 0.600 g/cm^2 and 1.000 g/cm^2, the cut-offs derived from CV vary between 0.015 g/cm^2 and 0.024 g/cm^2, 0.024 g/cm^2 and 0.041 g/cm^2, 0.018 g/cm^2 and 0.030 g/cm^2, 0.015 g/cm^2 and 0.025 g/cm^2 for the spine femoral neck, greater trochanter, and total hip, respectively. In postmenopausal osteoporotic women aged >70 years, for the same range of BMD level, cut-offs vary between 0.031 g/cm^2 and 0.051 g/cm^2, 0.038 g/cm^2 and 0.063 g/cm^2, 0.043 g/cm^2 and 0.071 g/cm^2, 0.038 g/cm^2 and 0.063 g/cm^2 for the same bone sites. Consequently, to express variability on a percentage basis using CV leads to underestimate variability in patients with low BMD and to overestimate variability in patients with high BMD. Previous reports in the literature, as well as Ravaud, Lodder's data and our data (table 1) demonstrate that absolute precision errors derived from SD are constant across a wide range of BMD values and independent of the level of BMD. Because of therapeutic consequences, the clinician should be especially careful in judging an apparent BMD change in patients with osteoporosis. Influence of age on BMD reproducibility is controversial. Previous studies have suggested that BMD measurement errors were independent of age even some studies suggested that SDD may vary in extreme ages (children and elderly) probably because of age-related factors other than BMD. However, a few data exist for reproducibility of DXA in women over 70. Ravaud et al. data, as well as those of Fuleihan (Fuleihan, Testa et al. 1995), and Maggio et al. (Maggio, McCloskey et al. 1998) show that the measurement error is greater in older osteoporotic subjects. Several factors such as difficulties in repositioning could explain the increase of measurement error in this kind of patients. Therefore, the use of the SDD in the evaluation of an apparent BMD change gives a more conservative approach than the use of the CV at low BMD. Because of its independence from the BMD level and its expression in absolute units, the SDD is a preferable measure for use in daily clinical practice as compared with the CV and the derived LSC.

In contrast with all previous publications about DXA reproducibility, we found in our centre better results for the hip BMD variability than the lumbar spine. This is due to the fact that our study was the first to use the mean measure of the two femurs (dual femur). In this study, we showed in a group of young healthy volunteers that the SDD was ±0.0218 g/cm^2 when both femurs were measured whereas it was ±0.0339 g/cm^2 when only one femur was measured. Thus, these results enhance to encourage the use of the measurement of both hips to improve the reproducibility of DXA at this site.

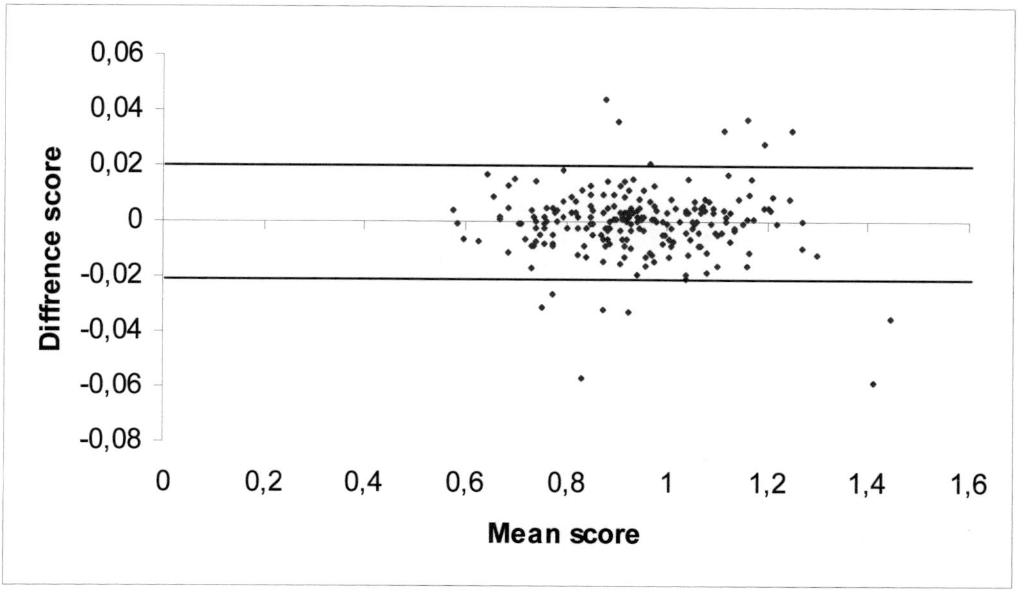

(a)

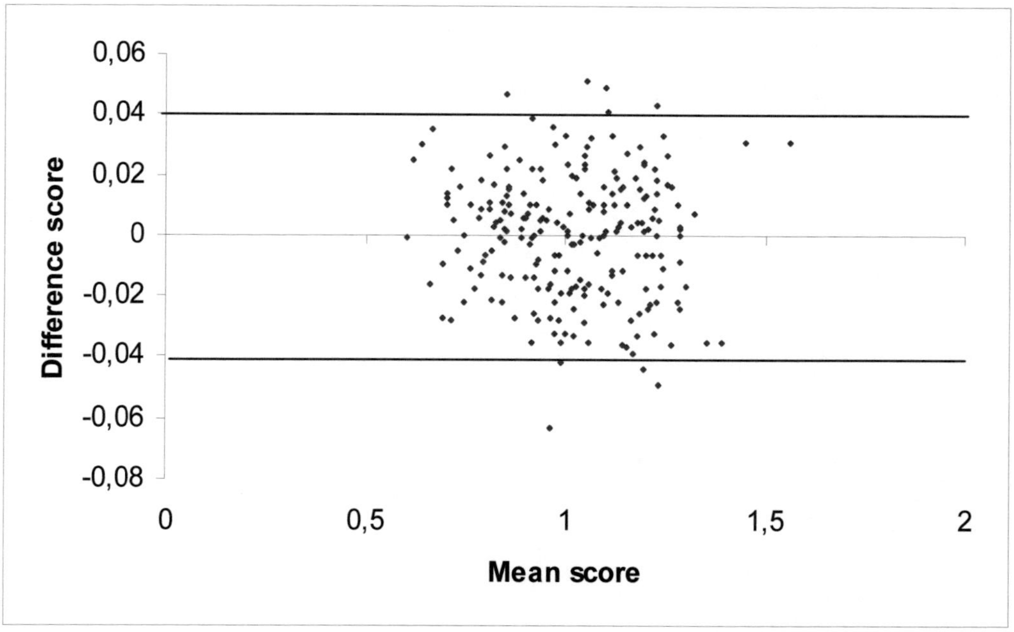

(b)

Fig. 1. Graph of the difference score against the mean score of the total hip (a) and the lumbar spine (b) BMD measurements (g/cm^2) in our centre [17] using Bland and Altman method. The outermost (solid) lines represent the SDD.

	El Maghraoui et al. [17]						Lodder et al. [9]			
	Healthy young volunteers n = 60 28.2 ± 5.5 years		Post menopausal women n = 102 58.1 ± 7.0 years		Chronic rheumatic diseases n= 60 47.1 ± 12.8 years		Post menopausal women n = 95 59.9 ± 8.1 years		Children n = 23 11.2 ± 1.3 years	
	LS	TH	LS	TH	LS	TH	LS	TH	LS	TH
Mean difference : m (SD) (systematic bias)	-0.0071 (±0.005)	-0.0001 (±0.003)	0.0015 (±0.004)	0.0006 (±0.002)	-0.0042 (±0.006)	0.0027 (±0.004)	-0.001 (±0.05)	-0.0004 (±0.04)	-0.0009 (±0.02)	-0.003 (±0.03)
SD (random measurement error)	0.0206	0.0111	0.0180	0.0109	0.0230	0.0146	0.0238	0.0184	0.0088	0.0116
SDD (g/cm²)	±0.0403	±0.0218	±0.0353	±0.0213	±0.0450	±0.0286	±0.0466	±0.0361	±0.0172	±0.0228
CV (%)	1.78	1.05	2.29	1.58	1.91	1.24	1.92	1.59	0.84	1.19
LSC (%)	4.94	2.90	6.35	4.38	5.29	3.44	5.43	4.50	2.38	3.37
Random effects ICC (95% CI)	0.98 (0.96 - 0.98)	0.99 (0.99 - 0.99)	0.99 (0.98 - 0.99)	0.99 (0.99 - 0.99)	0.99 (0.99 - 0.99)	0.99 (0.99 - 0.99)	0.99 (0.98 - 0.99)	0.99 (0.99 - 0.99)	0.99 (0.99 – 1.00)	0.99 (0.99 – 1.00)

Mean difference, mean of the difference between the first and the second BMD measurement; SD difference, SD of the difference between the first and the second BMD measurement; SDD, smallest detectable difference (g/cm^2); CV, coefficient of variation (%); LSC, least significant change (%); ICC, intraclass correlation coefficient.

Table 1. Comparison of BMD measurement reproducibility evaluation in two studies including various groups of patients.

Although the variability as expressed by the CV, and especially the SDD, is reassuring, showing good short term variability at group level, the wide range of the differences in BMD and the derived T-scores indicates considerable individual differences between two consecutive BMD measurements in some patients. The range in ΔT scores, for example, indicates that in some patients the diagnosis, based on the diagnostic thresholds of the WHO, would change owing to the measurement variability.

In summary, reproducibility of BMD measurement by DXA in different kinds of patients (postmenopausal women, patients with chronic rheumatic diseases, elderly…) expressed by different means is good at a group level. However, the clinician must remain aware that an apparent BMD change in an individual patient may represent a precision error. At each measurement centre, the SDD should be calculated from in vivo reproducibility data. In clinical practice, the SDD should be used to estimate the significance of observed changes, in absolute values.

5. Other factors influencing DXA monitoring

The first factor is the time interval between two measurements in the same patient which must be long enough to allow occurrence of a change greater than the SDD or the LSC. Therefore, it depends on the expected rate of change in BMD measurement (which varies according to whether the measurement site is composed predominantly of trabecular or of cortical bone) and the reproducibility of BMD measurement at that site. Thus, in clinical practice, a treatment-induced BMD increase can only be detected in general after 2 years. However, in patients receiving long term steroid therapy, the changes in BMD may be so important that they can be detected at 1 year. Thus, although the spine may not be the best site for the diagnosis of osteoporosis given the high prevalence of spinal degenerative disease, it is the most sensitive site for detecting changes over time. However, our study showed that measurement of both femurs (called "dual femur" in Lunar machines) increases the reproducibility at this site.

In another side, the changes in BMD measurements are influenced by the ability of osteoporosis treatments to increase the BMD at the different skeletal sites. For some treatments such as teriparatide and the more potent bisphosphonates, statistically significant changes in spine BMD occur on time scales of 1 to 2 years in the majority of patients, although for other treatments, such as raloxifene, the changes are often not large enough to be statistically significant. Recently, the strontium ranelate trials show BMD increases at the spine and hip 2-5 times larger than those for BPs and SERMs, and comparable or greater than with teriparatide. However, it is important to appreciate that much of this effect is due to the higher atomic number of strontium compared with calcium. Thus, strontium in bone attenuates X-rays much more strongly than calcium, and BMD is overestimated compared with the true mass of bone mineral present. This effect may persist for many years after the patient stops treatment and may affect the relationship between BMD and fracture risk.

Thus, treatment dosages cannot be adjusted on the basis of BMD changes. Moreover, there is no proof that repeating BMD measurements improves compliance, as most patients discontinue antiresorptive medications after a few months because of administration constraints, side effects, cost of medications or lack of interest.

Above all, BMD is used as a surrogate marker for the fracture risk, yet BMD increases do not reliably reflect a reduction in the fracture risk. Although bisphosphonates, raloxifene, and strontium have not been compared in the same study, they seem to produce comparable reductions in the risk of vertebral fractures, of about 30–50%, whereas BMD changes differ markedly across medications. Studies have shown that BMD gains explain only a small proportion of the vertebral fracture risk reduction: 28% with risedronate(Li, Meredith et al. 2001), 16% with alendronate(Cummings, Karpf et al. 2002), and 4% with raloxifene(Sarkar, Mitlak et al. 2002). It has been suggested that the percentage of BMD change may be related to the change in the relative risk of fracture(Wasnich and Miller 2000). In one study, a linear relationship was found between these two parameters, but a 1% increase in spinal BMD was associated with an only 3% decrease in the relative risk of vertebral fracture(Cummings, Karpf et al. 2002). For peripheral fractures, in contrast, the risk reduction is clearly related to the BMD gain(Hochberg, Greenspan et al. 2002). Common sense indicates that a BMD increase during treatment should be preferable over a BMD decrease. However, data showing that the fracture risk may decrease despite a reduction in BMD have been reported (Watts, Geusens et al. 2005). It has also been shown that the fracture risk was more heavily dependent on BMD at baseline than on BMD changes during treatment (Hochberg, Ross et al. 1999).

6. Conclusion

Serial BMD measurements can be used to monitor current antiresorptive treatments (raloxifene, bisphosphonates or strontium ranelate). However, adequate quality-control procedures must be used(Roux, Garnero et al. 2005). Measurement error must be considered when evaluating serial assessments. A clear understanding of the interpretation of serial measurements and the statistical principles impacting upon their interpretation is necessary to determine whether a change is real and not simply random fluctuation. It is inadequate to simply use the manufacturer's default precision error, which may underestimate the precision error in the clinical setting. Thus, every centre should calculate its own precision error from in vivo reproducibility data. International societies interested in osteoporosis diagnosis and management such as the International Society for Clinical Densitometry or the International Osteoporosis Foundation should add to their guidelines at least two recommendations about DXA monitoring highlighted in this paper: the measurement of both hips improves the reproducibility at this site and DXA measurement centres should determine and use the individual SDD. Indeed, the use of the SDD is preferable to the use of the CV and LSC because of its independence from BMD level and its expression in absolute units. The exact definition and advices for the measure and use of these parameters in clinical practice should be clearly explained. It is clear that the choice of the optimum site for performing follow-up scans depends on the ratio of the BMD treatment effect to the precision of the measurements. The larger this ratio, the more statistically significant the observed changes are likely to be. Actually, all data agree in showing that the spine is the optimum site. In clinical practice, BMD measurements have to be spaced at least 2 years apart. The main goal of serial BMD measurement is to check that no further bone loss has occurred; estimation of BMD gains is the secondary objective. This should be explained to the patients, many of whom expect to recover normal BMD values.

7. References

Bland, J. M. and D. G. Altman (1986). "Statistical methods for assessing agreement between two methods of clinical measurement." *Lancet* 1(8476): 307-10.

Cummings, S. R., D. B. Karpf, et al. (2002). "Improvement in spine bone density and reduction in risk of vertebral fractures during treatment with antiresorptive drugs." *Am J Med* 112(4): 281-9.

Eastell, R. (1996). "Assessment of bone density and bone loss." *Osteoporos Int* 6 Suppl 2: 3-5.

El Maghraoui, A. and C. Roux (2008). "DXA scanning in clinical practice." *QJM* 101(8): 605-17.

El Maghraoui, A., A. A. Do Santos Zounon, et al. (2005). "Reproducibility of bone mineral density measurements using dual X-ray absorptiometry in daily clinical practice." *Osteoporos Int* 16(12): 1742-8.

El Maghraoui, A., L. Achemlal, et al. (2006). "Monitoring of dual-energy X-ray absorptiometry measurement in clinical practice." *J Clin Densitom* 9(3): 281-6.

Fuleihan, G. E., M. A. Testa, et al. (1995). "Reproducibility of DXA absorptiometry: a model for bone loss estimates." *J Bone Miner Res* 10(7): 1004-14.

Gluer, C. C. (1999). "Monitoring skeletal changes by radiological techniques." *J Bone Miner Res* 14(11): 1952-62.

Gluer, C. C., G. Blake, et al. (1995). "Accurate assessment of precision errors: how to measure the reproducibility of bone densitometry techniques." *Osteoporos Int* 5(4): 262-70.

Hochberg, M. C., P. D. Ross, et al. (1999). "Larger increases in bone mineral density during alendronate therapy are associated with a lower risk of new vertebral fractures in women with postmenopausal osteoporosis. Fracture Intervention Trial Research Group." *Arthritis Rheum* 42(6): 1246-54.

Hochberg, M. C., S. Greenspan, et al. (2002). "Changes in bone density and turnover explain the reductions in incidence of nonvertebral fractures that occur during treatment with antiresorptive agents." *J Clin Endocrinol Metab* 87(4): 1586-92.

Johnson, S. L., V. I. Petkov, et al. (2005). "Improving osteoporosis management in patients with fractures." *Osteoporos Int* 16(9): 1079-85.

Li, Z., M. P. Meredith, et al. (2001). "A method to assess the proportion of treatment effect explained by a surrogate endpoint." *Stat Med* 20(21): 3175-88.

Lodder, M. C., W. F. Lems, et al. (2004). "Reproducibility of bone mineral density measurement in daily practice." *Ann Rheum Dis* 63(3): 285-9.

Maggio, D., E. V. McCloskey, et al. (1998). "Short-term reproducibility of proximal femur bone mineral density in the elderly." *Calcif Tissue Int* 63(4): 296-9.

Maillefert, J. F., L. S. Aho, et al. (2001). "Changes in bone density in patients with ankylosing spondylitis: a two-year follow-up study." *Osteoporos Int* 12(7): 605-9.

Nguyen, T. V., P. N. Sambrook, et al. (1997). "Sources of variability in bone mineral density measurements: implications for study design and analysis of bone loss." *J Bone Miner Res* 12(1): 124-35.

Phillipov, G., C. J. Seaborn, et al. (2001). "Reproducibility of DXA: potential impact on serial measurements and misclassification of osteoporosis." *Osteoporos Int* 12(1): 49-54.

Ravaud, P., J. L. Reny, et al. (1999). "Individual smallest detectable difference in bone mineral density measurements." *J Bone Miner Res* 14(8): 1449-56.

Roux, C., P. Garnero, et al. (2005). "Recommendations for monitoring antiresorptive therapies in postmenopausal osteoporosis." *Joint Bone Spine* 72(1): 26-31.

Sarkar, S., B. H. Mitlak, et al. (2002). "Relationships between bone mineral density and incident vertebral fracture risk with raloxifene therapy." *J Bone Miner Res* 17(1): 1-10.

Wasnich, R. D. and P. D. Miller (2000). "Antifracture efficacy of antiresorptive agents are related to changes in bone density." *J Clin Endocrinol Metab* 85(1): 231-6.

Watts, N. B., P. Geusens, et al. (2005). "Relationship between changes in BMD and nonvertebral fracture incidence associated with risedronate: reduction in risk of nonvertebral fracture is not related to change in BMD." *J Bone Miner Res* 20(12): 2097-104.

3

Bone Loss and Seasonal Variation in Serial DXA Densitometry – A Population-Based Study

Joonas Sirola[1,2], Toni Rikkonen[1], Risto Honkanen[1], Jukka S. Jurvelin[3], Marjo Tuppurainen[1,4] and Heikki Kröger[1,2],
[1]*University of Eastern Finland, Campus of Kuopio, Bone and Cartilage Research Unit*
[2]*Department of Orthopedics, Traumatology and Hand Surgery*
[3]*Department of Clinical Physiology & Nuclear Medicine*
[4]*Department of Obstetrics and Gynaecology*
[2,3,4]*Kuopio University Hospital, Finland*

1. Introduction

Osteoporosis is a disease of increased skeleton fragility accompanied by low BMD and microarchitectural deterioration. Osteoporosis and bone fragility result in significant morbidity and medical and social costs (Dennison et al., 2005; Cummings et al., 2002). The risk of fractures is greater among women with low BMD although it explains only part of the increased fracture tendency among the elderly (National Osteoporosis Foundation, 1998).The diagnosis of osteoporosis is currently based on axial dual X-ray absorptiometry (DXA) measurements (National Osteoporosis Foundation 1998). In addition to being applicable for fracture prediction, axial DXA has a role in treatment monitoring protocols (Miller et al., 1996; Sowers et al., 1997). Furthermore, serial central DXA measurements have been used for research purposes to evaluate the risk- and preventive factors for postmenopausal bone loss (Burger et al., 1998; Hannan et al., 2000; Sirola et al., 2003) Perimenopausal bone loss rates of over -2 percent /year in spinal and over -1 percent /year in the femoral region have generally been reported (Harris and Dawson-Hughes, 1992; Pouilles et al., 1993; Pouilles et al., 1995; Prior et al., 1998; Ito et al., 1999). In postmenopausal women, age related bone loss continues at age specific rate after the initial fastening during the menopausal transition (Hansen et al., 1995).

There are two forms of vitamin D, ergocalciferol (vitamin D2) and cholecalciferol (vitamin D3). Cholecalciferol is the metabolically active form of vitamin D. Vitamin D is produced with either the effect of ultraviolet B radiation or ingested with nutrition and the metabolically active form is produced in the kidneys. It has been suggested that there might be a seasonal variation in bone turnover as assessed with both BMD and biochemical markers (Rosen et al., 1994.; Storm et al., 1998; Rapuri et al., 2002). The sun-light related vitamin D production which varies according to season seems to contribute to this phenomenon (Rapuri et al., 2002; Dawson-Hughes et al., 1997). However, other studies have not demonstrated any such effect as measured either by BMD or by levels of bone marker compounds (Patel et al, 2001; Blumsohn et al., 2003). Consequently, the effect of the season when densitometry was performed on bone density is still unresolved. Furthermore, the role of a seasonal difference between two distant follow-up bone density measurements in postmenopausal bone loss has not been studied and thus, nothing is known about the effect of this phenomenon on treatment monitoring or other longitudinal data collection. If present, such seasonal variation could have significant effect on the evaluation of prospective data.

The purpose of the present study was to investigate the effect of densitometry season on early postmenopausal BMD and bone loss in a subset of 954 Finnish women selected from the population-based Osteoporosis Risk Factor and Prevention (OSTPRE)-study.

2. Subjects and methods

2.1 Study population

The study population was a randomly selected part of the prospective Kuopio Osteoporosis Risk Factor and Prevention (OSTPRE) study cohort. The OSTPRE cohort was established in 1989 and included all women born in 1932-1941 and who were resident in Kuopio Province, Finland (n=14 220). A postal inquiry including questions about health disorders, medications including HRT, gynaecologic history, nutritional habits, physical activity, life-style habits, and anthropometric information was sent to these women at baseline in 1989 (Honkanen et al, 1991). The 5-year (in 1994 follow-up questionnaires were sent to the 13 100 women who responded at baseline and responses were received from 11 954 at 5-year follow-up. The study protocol has been approved by the ethics committee of University of Kuopio and Kuopio University Hospital. Informed written consent from the participants was collected with the postal inquiries.

Of the 13 100 respondents in 1989, 11 055 (84.4 %) were willing to undergo DXA densitometry. A random sample of 2 362 women was selected for densitometry out of which 2025 women actually underwent the procedure during 1989-91. The questionnaire information was updated at the time of bone densitometry. In all, 1 873 women underwent both baseline (1989-91) and follow-up (1994-97) measurements and 1 551 of these had valid serial measurements for both lumbar spine and femoral neck (excluding severe bone deformities, see section *Bone mass measurements*).

For the present study, the following women were additionally excluded: 1) hysterectomized women (for whom it was impossible to define the menopausal status) and bilaterally ovariectomized women (n=445), 2) premenopausal women (n=152). Accordingly, the final study population consisted of 954 women (beginning of menopause either before or during follow-up) aged 48 to 59 years at baseline densitometry. The beginning of menopause was defined as 12 months' amennorhea (WHO Scientific Group, 1996) and the duration of menopause varied from 1 to 26 years at follow-up densitometry. The duration of follow-up varied from 3.8 to 7.9 years (mean 5.8 years).

2.2 Seasonal Difference Index (SDI)

The study population was divided into three equal groups within the year according to month of measurement at baseline and follow-up: Group 1 (from January to April), Group 2 (from May to August) and Group 3 (from September to December). The basis for selecting these cut-offs was based on the assumption that highest BMDs (reflecting serum vitamin D concentration) would be present at late summer and early fall season (within group 2) and the lowest at late winter (within group 3) whereas group 1 would present an intermediate. Also, in order to reveal the greatest differences in seasonal BMD variation between two successive measurements a numeric value of a Seasonal Difference Index (SDI) was calculated as follows:

SDI = (Group number at baseline - Group number at follow-up)

Accordingly, the numeric value of SDI varied from -2 to +2 (Table 1). In all, 521 (54.6 %) women were measured within the same season at both measurements (SDI group 0). In 212 (22.2 %) women the follow-up measurement was carried out in a later season (SDI groups -1 and -2) and in 221 (23.2 %) women in earlier season (SDI groups +1 and +2) than the baseline measurement. There was a significant variation in distribution of women into measurement seasons between and within baseline and follow-up measurements (Figure 1). Accordingly, any conclusions over differences between specific seasons were considered to be precluded due to this uneven distribution.

	Follow-up season (Group number)		
Baseline season (Group number)	January-April (1)	May-August (2)	September-December (3)
January-April (1)	0	-1	-2
May-August (2)	1	0	-1
September-December (3)	2	1	0

a) SDI=[Season Group at baseline]-[Season Group at follow-up]

Table 1. Numeric values for the "Seasonal Difference Index" (SDI)[a] according to baseline and follow-up DXA measurement season

2.3 Other variables

2.3.1 Hormone therapy

Women were divided into two groups according to their use of hormone therapy (HRT) (tablets and plasters) which was defined as the use of hormonal products for menopausal symptoms. *HRT users* (n=393) had used HRT continuously or occasionally during the follow-up regardless of whether or not they had used hormonal therapy before the baseline (14 women used HRT only before baseline, and were excluded in analysis on HRT effect). *HRT non-users* (n=547) had never used estrogen containing products aimed at postmenopausal therapy. In the OSTPRE cohort, the majority of HRT users were taking estrogen-progesterone combination products (56.2% of all HRT). No data was available on whether HRT was continuous or sequential. Forty-five percent of HRT users (occasional or continuous) had been treated with HRT also prior to baseline. The duration of HRT varied from one month to 7.5 years. The information about the use of hormonal products was obtained from the questionnaires. Comparison between self-reported use of HRT and the national prescription records of The Social Insurance Institution, Finland (KELA), for the whole OSTPRE cohort in 1996–2001 revealed that 97.8% of those who had received an oestrogen drug prescription reported HRT use in inquiries. On the other hand, in 25.5% of the self-reported non-users of HRT some oestrogen use (short-term, median 6.0 months) was recorded (Sirola et al., 2003a).

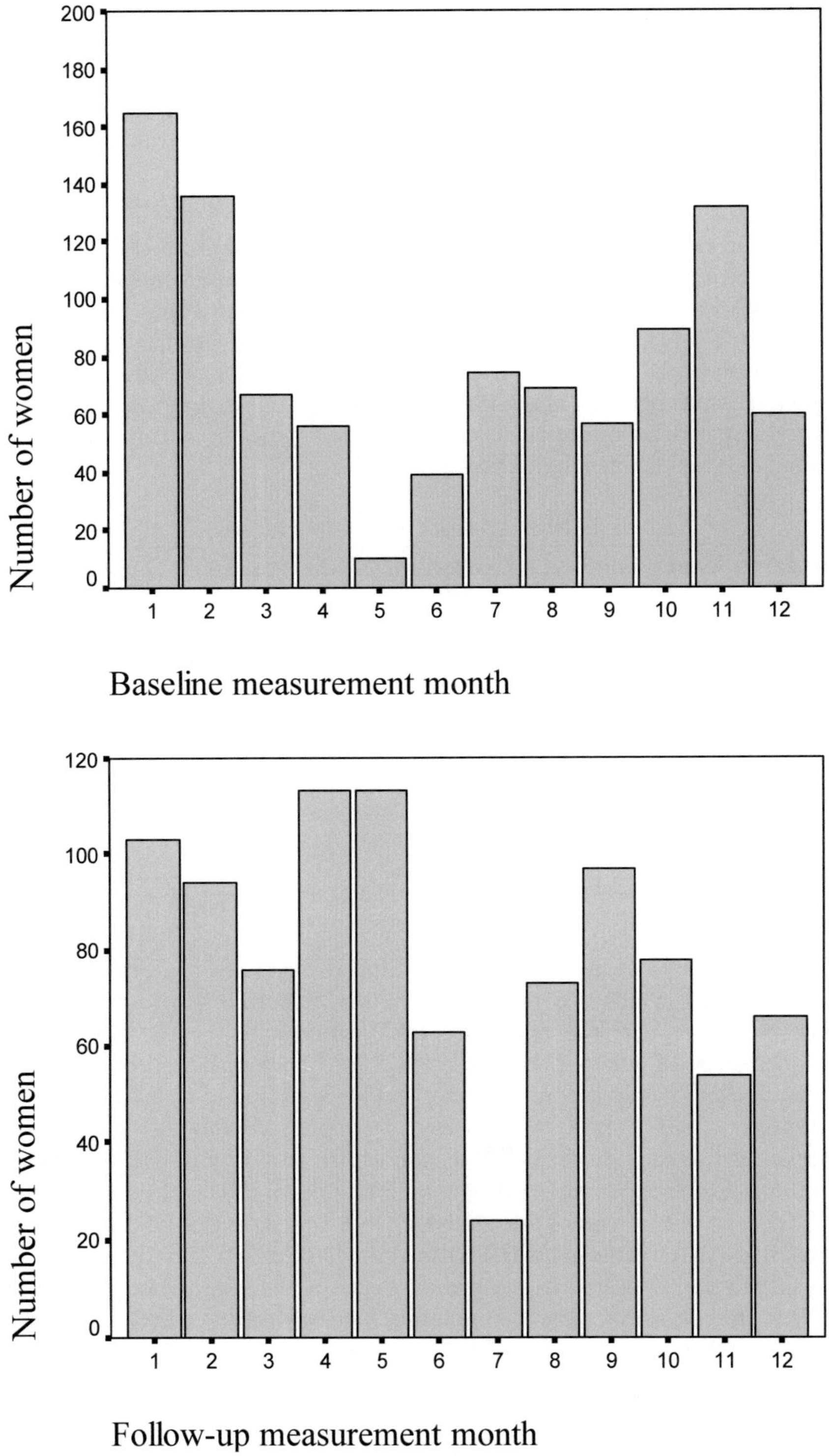

Fig. 1. Distribution of the study population accroding to DXA measurement month.

2.3.2 Adjusting variables

The *height* and *weight* were measured with a stadiometer and calibrated scale by study group nurses at each bone densitometry.

Nutritional calcium intake of each participant was estimated according to self-reported ingestion of milk products in postal inquiries. The following questions were asked:" How many deciliters of fluid milk products (milk, sour milk, yoghurt, etc.) do you consume daily? " and "How many slices of cheese do you eat daily?". The amount of calcium was approximated to be 120 mg/dl for fluid milk products and 87 mg/slice for cheese (Sirola et al., 2003b).

Women were divided into two categories (yes, no) according to the presence/absence of *bone affecting diseases or medications* at baseline. Bone affecting diseases/medications have been described previously by Kröger et al. (Kröger et al. 1994). Diseases were: renal disease, liver disease, insulin-dependent diabetes, malignancies, rheumatoid arthritis, endocrine abnormalities (parathyroid/thyroid glands, adrenals), malabsorption (including lactose malabsorption), total/partial gastrectomy, postovariectomy status, premenopausal amenorrhea, alcoholism and long-term immobilisation. Medications were: corticosteroids, diuretics, cytotoxic drugs, anticonvulsive drugs, anabolic steroids, calcitonin, bisphosphonates, vitamin D.

Physical activity level was calculated based on combined physical activity in work and leisure based on self-reports in the postal inquiries. The physical activity was categorised into low, moderate and high (Kröger et al., 1994).

2.4 Bone mass measurements

The bone mineral density of lumbar spine (L2-L4) and left femoral neck was determined using the same dual X-ray absorptiometry (DXA) (Lunar DPX, Madison, Wisconsin, USA) equipment at both the baseline and five year measurements. The measurements were carried out in Kuopio University Hospital by specially trained personnel. The short term reproducibility of this method has been shown to be 0.9 % for lumbar spine and 1.5 % for femoral neck BMD measurements (Kröger et al., 1992).The long-term reproducibility (coefficient of variation) of the DXA instrument for BMD during the study period, as determined by regular phantom measurements, was 0.4 % (Komulainen et al., 1998). Each DXA measurement print was reviewed and women with bone deformities (osteoarthritis, osteophytes, scoliosis and compression fractures) in either area were excluded from the analyses. At the time of densitometry, also the weight and height of each participant was measured in a controlled situation.

2.5 Statistical methods

Statistical analyses were carried out with the Statistical Package for Social Sciences (SPSS) for Windows, version 17. The annual BMD changes for both measurement sites were calculated as follows: [(BMD at the 5-year follow-up - BMD at baseline) / duration of follow-up in years] and reported as percentage of baseline BMD. In categorical analyses, uni- and multivariate analysis of variance was used and Tukey (crude models) and Least Significant Difference (adjusted models) -post hoc tests were utilized to study differences between multiple groups when applicable. Adjustment for age, height, weight, months since menopause, mean calcium intake, use of HRT (no, occasional, continuous), physical activity level (low, moderate, high), duration of follow-up (years) and the use of bone affecting medications or diseases (yes/no) (including vitamin D supplements) as covariates was performed.

3. Results

The baseline data revealed that there were no significant differences between the three season groups with respect to age, duration of menopause or HRT use (Table 2). There were no differences in the cross-sectional BMD between the season groups at baseline or at the five year follow-up (Table 2).

In order to evaluate a possible contribution of seasonal differences to the follow-up BMD values, the association of SDI with mean annual bone loss was investigated (Figure 2). The bone loss rate in SDI categories -2 and 0 was greater than in SDI categories +1 and +2 (p<0.01) in both lumbar and femoral regions (Figure 2). In lumbar spine, the difference in bone loss rate between SDI categories -1 and +1 was also significant (p=0.015). In femoral neck there was no significant difference between SDI category -1 and the other categories. These effects were independent of any adjustments.

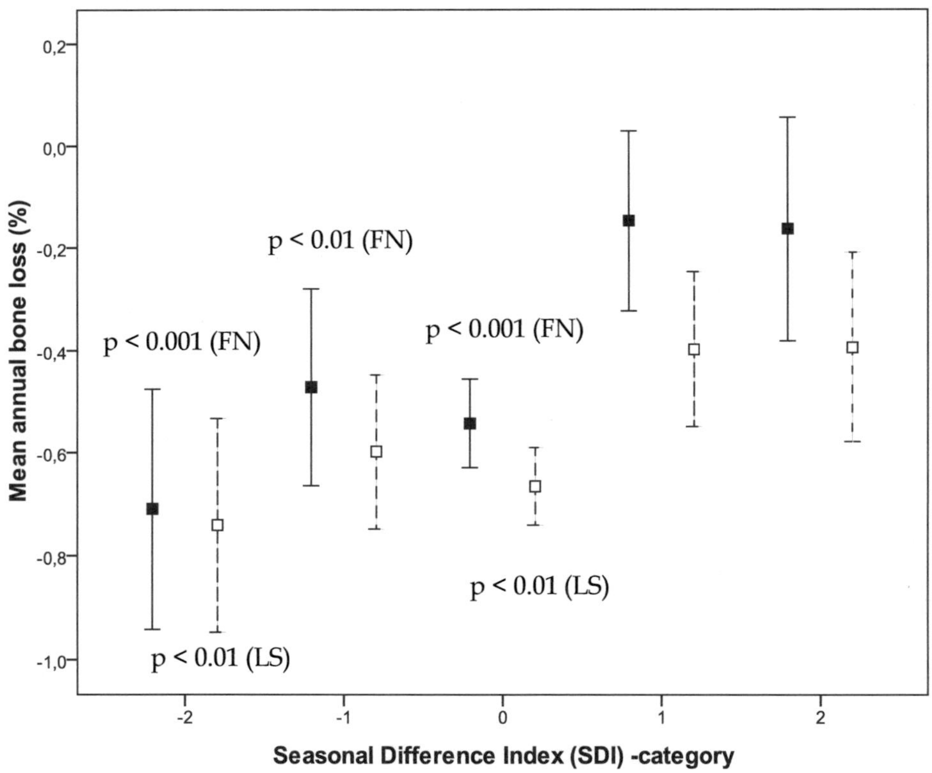

p-values refer to the differences of the respective SDI group in comparison to SDI 1 and 2 for lumbar spine (LS=full line) and femoral neck (FN=dotted line). a) adjusted for age, height, weight, months since menopause, calcium intake, use of HT (no, occasional, continuous), overall physical activity level (low, moderate, high), duration of follow-up (years) and use of bone affecting medications or diseases (yes/no)

Fig. 2. Effect of Seasonal Difference Index (SDI) on mean annual bone loss rate (%) in early postmenopausal women (n=954). Analysis of covariance[a]

Variable	Season group[a]			
	Group 1	Group 2	Group 3	Total
	(n=424)	(n=192)	(n=338)	(n=954)
Means (SD) of continuous variables				
Duration of follow-up yrs	5,9(0,5)	5,8(0,4)	5,8(0,5)	5,8 (0,5)
Duration of menopause, months	89,4(54,1)	86,2(48,1)	106,6(50,4)	95,0(52,3)[d]
Baseline age, yrs	53,5(3,0)	53,5(2,9)	54,2(2,7)	53,7(2,9)[d]
Baseline height, cm	160,9(5,1)	161,6(5,5)	160,8(5,3)	161,0(5,3)
Baseline weight, kg	69,1(12,4)	68,6(11,4)	69,3(11,9)	69,1(12,0)
Weight change (%)	2,9(5,2)	2,9(5,6)	3,0(5,3)	2,9(5,3)
Grip strength, kPa	62,0(16,5)	62,2(15,6)	62,4(16,0)	62,2(16,1)
Mean calcium intake, mg/day	789(343)	813(311)	799(319)	797(328)
Baseline lumbar BMD, g/cm^2	1,13(0,17)	1,13(0,16)	1,11(0,16)	1,12(0,16)
Baseline femoral neck BMD, g/cm^2	0,93(0,13)	0,93(0,13)	0,92(0,12)	0,92(0,13)
FU lumbar BMD, g/cm^2	1,07(0,17)	1,09(0,15)	1,07(0,16)	1,08(0,16)
FU femoral neck BMD, g/cm^2	0,88(0,12)	0,90(0,13)	0,89(0,12)	0,89(0,12)
B. Distribution of category variables (%)				
Use of HRT during follow-up				
No use	55,8	56,0	64,7	59,0 [c]
Occasional (<90 % of FU)	32,2	34,6	28,2	31,2
Continuous (>90 % of FU)	12,1	9,4	7,2	9,8
No bone affecting disease/medication	60,4	64,1	64,7	62,7
Any previous fracture at baseline	20,9	23,3	20,6	21,3
Previous wrist fracture at baseline	7,2	7,7	5,5	6,7
Alcohol >1 drink/week	35,1	34,4	32,3	33,9
Smoking	9,4	11,1	8,8	9,5
High overall physical activity level[b]	29,9	37,8	32,8	32,5

a) Season Groups: Group 1 (from January to April), Group 2 (from May to August) and Group 3 (from September to December). b) Three categorical variable: low, moderate, high. c) p<0.05 / d) p<0.001

Table 2. Baseline characteristics of the study population according to season group[a] (n=954).

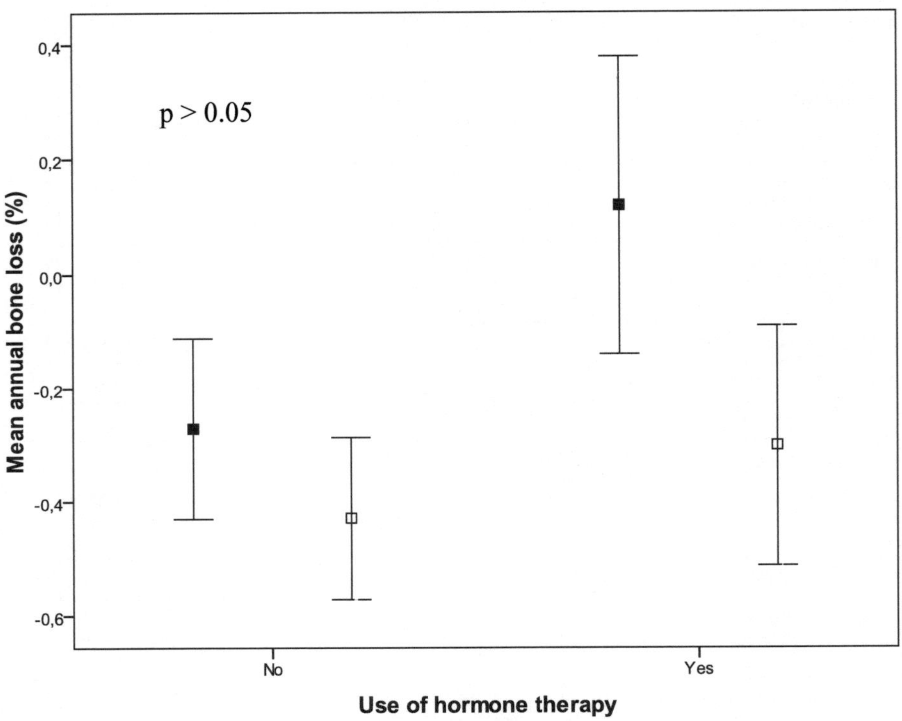

A: SDI category -2 to 0

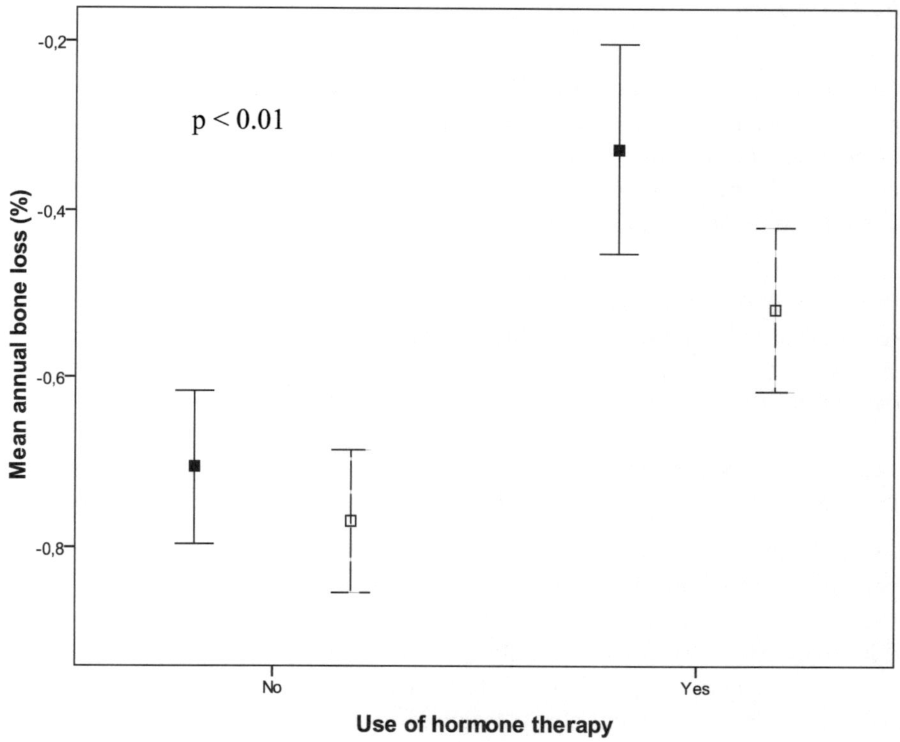

B: SDI category 1 and 2

Fig. 3. Effect of hormone therapy on lumbar spine (full line) and femoral neck (dotted line) bone loss according to seaosal difference index (SDI) category. Analysis of variance (ANOVA, n=954).

In ANOVA, SDI explained 2.3 percent (R^2=0.023) and 1.3 percent (R^2=0.013) of the bone mass changes in lumbar spine and femoral neck, respectively. Furthermore, in linear regression models, SDI was positively associated with both lumbar spine and femoral neck bone loss ($p<0.001$) independent of all adjustments.

In order to mimic the possible effect of SDI on a treatment monitoring protocol, we investigated the effects of HRT on bone loss according to SDI (Figure 3). HRT users had significantly lower bone loss rate in SDI categories -2 to 0 in comparison to HRT non-users (lumbar spine and femoral neck) ($p<0.01$). In SDI categories 1 to 2, there was no statistically significant difference between HRT users and non-users. These results were not affected by adjustments.

4. Discussion

The present study evaluated the effect of season on BMD and bone loss with a randomly selected population-based sample of 954 Finnish women. The seasonal difference between two successive axial DXA measurements, estimated with the "Seasonal Difference Index" (SDI), influenced the evaluation of postmenopausal bone loss rate. In addition, this factor interfered with the evaluation of protective bone effects of HRT. The exact direction of these relationships, in terms of specific seasons, was found to complex partly due to the study setting.

The present study sample was large and randomly selected. There were few differences in the baseline variables between the three season groups. The DXA measurements were carried out with same equipment and measurement staff and all bone deformities were excluded. In addition, phantom calibration was performed regularly which should exclude any significant seasonal changes attributable to equipment performance. Furthermore, comprehensive adjustment for any potential confounders was used in the analyses. Hence, it is most unlikely that any major confounding could have occurred in the present study.

Some weaknesses of the present study should also be considered. The follow-up time was relatively long with considerable inter-individual variation. Although the results were adjusted for duration of follow-up and reported in annual percent changes the follow-up period in treatment monitoring is usually only one or two years. However, the long follow-up and large sample probably facilitated the detection of bone mass changes in the present study. Furthermore, the present study assumed that the pattern of bone loss between the approximately five-year follow-up was linear, masking any possible short-term non-linear patterns. However, adjusting for these changes would have required DXA measurement at the very least at 1 year intervals. Lastly, the lack of information of serum vitamin D levels precluded causal conclusions. However, adjustment for bone affecting medication (including vitamin D containing products, medications and supplements) and calcium intake was performed eliminating bias due to these factors.

The results of the present study have two major applications. Firstly, in treatment monitoring, an attempt should be made to measure bone density within the same season. Naturally, the seasonal limits depend on amount of seasonal variation in sunlight exposure of the study population and should be closely studied. The sub-division used in the present study provides one example in DXA measurements suitable for Scandinavian latitudes.

Secondly, in prospective studies, possible distortion in results due to seasonal differences in risk-factor analyses and treatment effects on bone loss rate should be closely considered. Accordingly, it could be worthwhile to create a "seasonal difference index" for each population based on the respective DXA measurement data. The effect of seasonal differences on densitometry-based risk-factors for postmenopausal bone loss remains to be resolved. It might be that seasonal dependency could interact with certain factors lessening their true impacts. Also, the impact of these differences on fracture prediction remains to be resolved in future studies.

The interpretation of seasonal indices needs to be undertaken with caution. In the present study, the differences between the SDI categories do not necessarily provide information of the exact season that each participant was measured (e.g. SDI +1 could represent a difference between baseline season category 3 and a 5-year season category 2 or a baseline category 2 and a 5-year category 1). Also, the baseline and follow-up season groups (groups 1, 2, 3) itself included quite heterogeneous population. For example, the women measured during the first months of group 1 (January-February) were likely to have significantly lower BMDs in comparison to women presenting the other end (March-April) during which sun light exposure would be higher. We used this season categorisation order to categorize the measurement months into three equal groups within a year (i.e. four months per group: Spring (January-April), Summer (May-August) and Fall/Winter (September-December). This was based on the rapid changes in sun light exposure in the northern latitudes: sun light hours rapidly increase during may and decrease rapidly during september. Furthermore, the distribution of women into measurement months within each group was found to differ between baseline and follow-up densitometry. However, the goal of the present study was not to identify specific "risk seasons", but only to assess variability in the estimated bone loss rate attributable to the seasons when the two successive measurements had been done. Thus, some arbitrary cut-offs, in terms of season groups, were forced to be decided. Accordingly, the hypothesis of high or low bone density according to sun exposure (and vitamin D levels) in baseline and follow-up was precluded by skew distribution of women into different measurement months. Before adaptation for wider use, these indices would need further testing and refinement in order to optimize the categorisation for local purposes.

This is the first long-term population-based study investigating the contribution of seasonal difference between two successive DXA measurements on postmenopausal bone loss. Previous studies have shown significant alterations in vitamin D and PTH levels attributable to season (Rapuri et al., 2002; Dawson-Hughes et al., 1997).which could also provide a pathophysiological mechanism for the seasonal bone effects. Some studies have also found seasonal variation in cross-sectional BMD data, bone markers and bone loss rate (Rosen et al., 1994.; Storm et al., 1998; Rapuri et al., 2002; Dawson-Hughes et al., 1997). However, other studies have failed to found any evidence on altered bone metabolism related to seasons as measured with either BMD or bone markers (Patel et al, 2001; Blumsohn et al., 2003). The ability to observe seasonal effects is likely to depend on geographical location. Another study conducted in northern latitudes (Gerdhem et al, 2004) failed to demonstrate any seasonal variation in cross-sectional study design in Sweden. The present large study population, living at northern latitudes (latitude 63 degrees), might facilitate the detection of seasonal differences. However, the present study also showed no significant cross-sectional variation in BMD.

The present study also attempted to evaluate the possible bias in treatment monitoring resulting from seasonal difference via an investigation of how the SDI could affect the bone effect of HRT. In fact, variability in the protective effect of HRT between the SDI groups was detected. This serves as preliminary example of the extensiveness of the distortion in estimation of bone loss rate caused by seasonal difference. The inclusion of occasional use of HRT and less-than-perfect validity of HRT use in "non-users" probably mdified the results (Sirola et al., 2003a) but the trend was clear. Also, the effects may have been affected by lack of power due to small group sizes. However, seasonal densitometry difference may help in the identification of "non-responders" to HRT and be included in the list of other contributing factors (Sirola et al., 2003c; Komulainen et al., 1999). Previously, it has been suggested that calcium may flatten the seasonal differences in bone loss rate among elderly women[8] and that there might be seasonal variation in the bone response to vitamin D (Dawson-Hughes et al, 1991). The present study also showed abolition in the difference in the bone loss rate between SDI categories in HRT users.

In summary, seasonal differences should receive closer attention in treatment monitoring protocols and longitudinal risk factor studies. In future studies, the seasonal densitometry difference should be considered as a potential confounder and its effect on risk factor and treatment monitoring data should be assessed. In addition, factors that might lessen the seasonal changes in the bone loss rate, such as calcium, vitamin D and other bone drugs, should be identified. Our study raises, for the first time, the question of whether the results of longitudinal DXA measurements might be significantly distorted by seasonal differences especially in northern latitudes.

5. Acknowledgements

This work has been financially supported by Kuopio University Hospital, EVO-grant

6. References

Blumsohn A, Naylor KE, Timm W, Eagleton AC, Hannon RA, Eastell R (2003) Absence of marked seasonal change in bone turnover: a longitudinal and multicenter cross-sectional study. *J Bone Miner Res* 18:1274-1281

Burger H, de Laet CE, van Daele PL, Weel AE, Witteman JC, Hofman A, Pols HA (1998) Risk factors for increased bone loss in an elderly population: the Rotterdam Study. *Am J Epidemiol* 147:871-9.

Cummings SR, Melton LJ (2002) Epidemiology and outcomes of osteoporotic fractures. *Lancet* 359:1761–1767

Dawson-Hughes B, Dallal GE, Krall EA, Harris S, Sokoll LJ, Falconer G (1991) Effects of vitamin D supplementation on wintertime and overall bone loss in healthy postmenopausal women. *Ann Intern Med* 115:505-12

Dawson-Hughes B, Harris SS, Dallal GE (1997) Plasma calcidiol, season and serum parathyroid hormone concentration in healthy elderly men and women. *Am J Clin Nutr* 65:67-71

Dennison E, Cole Z, Cooper C (2005) Diagnosis and epidemiology of osteoporosis. *Curr Opin Rheumatol* 17(4):456–461

Gerdhem P, Mallmin H, Akesson K, Obrant KJ. Seasonal variation in bone density in postmenopausal women. *J Clin Densitom* 2004;7(1):93-100

Hannan MT, Felson DT, Dawson-Hughes B, Tucker KL, Cupples LA, Wilson PW, Kiel DP (2000) Risk factors for longitudinal bone loss in elderly men and women: the Framingham osteoporosis study. *J Bone Miner Res* 15:710-720.

Hansen MA, Overgaard K, Christiansen C (1995) Spontaneous postmenopausal bone loss in different skeletal areas followed up for 15 years. *J Bone Miner Res* 10:205-210

Harris S, Dawson-Hughes B (1992) Rates of change in bone mineral density of spine, heel, femoral neck and radius in healthy postmenopausal women. *Bone Miner* 17:87-95

Honkanen R, Tuppurainen M, Alhava E, Saarikoski S (1991) Kuopio Osteoporosis Risk Factor and Prevention Study. Baseline postal inquiry in 1989. *Publications of the University of Kuopio, Community Health, Statistics and Reviews 3/1991*; Kuopio.

Ito M, Nakamura T, Tsurusaki K, Uetani M, Hayashi K (1999) Effects of menopause on age-dependent bone loss in the axial and appendicular skeletons in healthy Japanese women. *Osteoporos Int* 19:377-83.

Komulainen MH, Kröger H, Tuppurainen MT, Heikkinen A-M, Alhava E, Honkanen R, Saarikoski S (1998) HRT and vit D in prevention of non-vertebral fractures in postmenopausal women; a 5 year randomised trial. *Maturitas* 31:45-54

Komulainen MH, Kröger H, Tuppurainen MT, Heikkinen A-M, Alhava E, Honkanen R, Jurvelin J, Saarikoski S (1999) Prevention of femoral and lumbar bone loss with hormone replacement therapy and vitamin D3 in early postmenopausal women: a population-based 5-year randomised trial. *J Clin Endoc Metab* 84:546-552

Kröger H, Heikkinen J, Laitinen K, Kotaniemi A (1992) Dual-energy X-ray absorptiometry in normal women: a cross-sectional study of 717 Finnish volunteers. *Osteoporos Int* 2:135-140.

Kröger H, Tuppurainen M, Honkanen R, Alhava E, Saarikoski S (1994) Bone mineral density and risk factors for osteoporosis-a population based study of 1600 perimenopausal women. *Calcif Tissue Int* 55:1-7

Miller PD, Bonnick SL, Rosen CJ (1996) Consensus of an international panel on the clinical utility of bone mass measurements in the detection of low bone mass in the adult population. *Calcif Tissue Int* 58:207-214

National Osteoporosis Foundation (1998) Osteoporosis: review of the evidence for prevention, diagnosis, and treatment and cost-effectiveness analysis-status report. *Osteoporosis Int* 18 (suppl 4):S1-S88

Patel R, Collins D, Bullock S, Swaminathan R, Blake GM, Fogelman I (2001) The effect of season and vitamin D supplementation on bone mineral density in healthy women: a double-masked crossover study. *Osteoporos Int* 12:319-25

Pouilles JM, Tremollieres F, Ribot C (1993) The effects of menopause on longitudinal bone loss from the spine. *Calcif Tissue Int* 52:340-343

Pouilles JM, Tremollieres F, Ribot C (1995) Effect of menopause on femoral and vertebral bone loss. *J Bone Miner Res* 10:1531-1536

Prior JC (1998) Perimenopause: the complex endocrinology of the menopausal transition. *Endoc Res* 19(4):397-428

Rapuri PB, Kinyamu HK, Gallagher JC, Haynatzka V (2002) Seasonal changes in calcitropic hormones, bone markers and bone mineral density in elderly women. *J Clin Endocrinol Metab* 87:2024-32

Rosen CJ, Morrison A, Zhou H, Storm D, Hunter SJ, Musgrave K, Chen T, Wei W, Holick MF (1994) Elderly women in northern New England exhibit seasonal changes in bone mineral density and calciotropic hormones. *Bone Miner* 25:83-92

Sirola J, Kröger H, Honkanen R, Sandini L, Tuppurainen M, Jurvelin JS, Saarikoski S (2003a) Risk factors associated with peri- and postmenopausal bone loss - does HRT prevent weight loss- related bone loss? *Osteoporosis Int* 14: 27-33

Sirola J, Kröger H, Honkanen R, Jurvelin JS, Sandini L, Tuppurainen M, Saarikoski S (2003b) Smoking may impair the bone protective effects of nutritional calcium- a population based approach. *J Bone Miner Res* 18: 1036-1043

Sirola J, Kröger H, Jurvelin JS, Sandini L, Tuppurainen M, Saarikoski S, Honkanen R (2003c) Interaction of nutritional calcium and HRT in prevention of postmenopausal bone loss: a prospective study. *Calcif Tissue Int* 72:659-665

Sowers MF (1997) Clinical epidemiology and osteoporosis. Measures and their interpretation. *Endocrin Metab North Amer* 26:219-231

Storm D, Eslin R, Porter ES, Musgrave K, Vereault D, Patton C, Kessenich C, Mohan S, Chen T, Holick MF, Rosen CJ (1998) Calcium supplementation prevents seasonal bone loss and changes in biochemical markers of bone turnover in elderly New England women: a randomized placebo-controlled trial. *J Clin Endocrinol Metab* 83:3817-25

WHO Scientific Group (1996) Research on the menopause in the 1990's. *A report of the WHO Scientific Group*. World Health Organisation, Geneva, Switzerland, vol 866:1-79.

Part 2

Body Composition

4

The Validity of Body Composition Measurement Using Dual Energy X-Ray Absorptiometry for Estimating Resting Energy Expenditure

Chiyoko Usui[1,2], Motoko Taguchi[3],
Kazuko Ishikawa-Takata[4] and Mitsuru Higuchi[5]
[1]*Department of Health Promotion and Exercise,*
National Institute of Health and Nutrition,
[2]*Research Fellow of the Japan Society for the Promotion of Science,*
[3]*Japan Women's College of Physical Education,*
[4]*Department of Nutritional Education,*
National Institute of Health and Nutrition,
[5]*Faculty of Sport Sciences, Waseda University,*
Japan

1. Introduction

Tissue energy production varies over time, and for practical purposes, can be organized into three main components, resting energy expenditure (REE), the thermic effect of food, and the thermic effect of physical activity (Ravussin & Bogardus, 1989). To maintain body weight, energy from food intake must equal energy expenditure. The energy requirement is defined as the average dietary energy intake that is predicted to maintain energy balance in healthy adults of a given age, gender, weight, height, and level of physical activity consistent with good health, and can be estimated from REE. REE reflects underlying tissue composition, mass, and metabolic activity (Elia, 1992) and accounts for 60–80% of total daily energy expenditure compared with the thermic effects of feeding and physical activity (~10% and ~15-30%, respectively). The REE has a large impact on the regulation of body mass and energy balance. In the field of obesity research, the presence and genesis of between-individual REE differences is a topic of great interest. To date, some earlier studies demonstrated that body mass, especially fat-free mass (FFM), has been a useful candidate in estimating REE (Ravussin & Bogardus, 1989; Fukagawa et al., 1990; Tataranni & Ravussin, 1995). Therefore, it is important to accurately evaluate REE and to measure body composition by methods that are practical, precise, and accurate.

A strategy for exploring between-individual differences in REE is to apply a tissue organ prediction model (Elia, 1992; Wang et al., 2000; Gallagher et al., 1998 & 2000). Each tissue and organ mass is quantified using either computed tomography (CT) or magnetic resonance imaging (MRI), and assigned assumed specific resting metabolic rates (Elia, 1992). The product of tissue organ mass and specific resting metabolic rate is then taken as the tissue organ REE, with the sum representing total body REE.

$$REE = k_1 \times \text{tissue organ mass}_1 + k_2 \times \text{tissue organ mass}_2 + k_3 \times \text{tissue organ mass}_3 + \cdots$$

Dual-energy X-ray absorptiometry (DXA) can easily and accurately assess the body composition, including bone mineral content (BMC), fat mass (FM), and lean soft tissue mass (LST) of the whole body and the segments (Mazes et al., 1990; Svendsen et al., 1991 & 1993). In addition, recent studies support the use of DXA as a means of providing a "metabolic map" for exploring between individual or group differences in observed REE values (Hunter et al., 2001; Hayes et al., 2002; Usui et al., 2009). Specifically, the LST of the arms and legs, as provided by regional DXA estimates, represents primarily low-metabolic rate skeletal muscle tissue. In contrast, LST of the head and trunk includes all of the tissue organs with high metabolic rates, such as brain, heart, liver, kidneys, spleen, and gastrointestinal tract. Total body-fat estimates reflect low metabolic rate adipose tissue. The various regional and whole-body estimates thus provide a qualitative metabolic body composition map of high and low metabolic rate components. Hayes et al. (2002) demonstrated that REE can be estimated from five measured DXA values: body weight, total body fat mass, bone mineral content, appendicular lean mass, and head area. Their study showed that no bias was detected between measured and predicted REEs (Hayes et al., 2002). These results were quite good and support the overall concept that predictable relations exist between major tissue organ level components and heat production at rest. In view of the finding of Hayes et al. (2002), we improved the estimation model from the five component model to four component model (adipose tissue, skeletal muscle, bone, and residual tissue organs). It was also evaluated the possibility that measurement of the magnitude and distribution of fundamental somatic heat-producing units using DXA can be used to estimate REE in both young and elderly women with different aerobic fitness levels (Usui et al., 2009). We suggested that REE in adult women can be estimated from four tissue organ components by using DXA regardless of age and aerobic fitness levels.

On the other hand, the traditional REE estimation approach, now widely applied, is to link REE with body composition determinants using a two-compartment model consisting of FM and FFM (Wang et al., 2000). Empirical regression models are developed with REE set as the dependent variable, and age, race, sex, height, and weight (FFM and FM) set as potential predictor variables. The Harris–Benedict equation (Harris & Benedict, 1919), Schofield equation (Schofield, 1985), and the Food and Agriculture Organization of the United Nations/World Health Organization/United Nations University (FAO/WHO/UNU) equation (FAO/WHO/UNU, 1985) are internationally used. In Japan, Dietary Reference Intakes for Japanese (DRI (Japan)) provides basal metabolic rate (BMR ≒ REE) standards according to sex and age categories (Ministry of Heaith, Labour and Welfare of Japan, 2009). REE can be calculated as BMR standards multiplied by body weight. In addition, Ganpule et al. (2007) recently developed new predictive equations (NIHN (Japan)) for REE in Japanese.

In the present chapter, we evaluated the validity of body composition measurement using DXA for estimating REE. The REEs which are predicted by the equations of Harris-Benedict, Schofield, FAO/WHO/UNU, DRI (Japan), and NIHN (Japan) will then be cross-validated against our measured and predicted values by using DXA.

2. Body composition analysis

2.1 Anthropometric measurements

Body weight (BW) was measured to the nearest 0.1 kg by using an electronic scale (Inner Scan; Tanita Co., Japan and UC-321; A&D Co., Ltd., Tokyo, Japan), and height (Ht) was measured to thenearest 0.1cm by using a stadiometer (YL-65 and ST-2M; Yagami Inc., Japan). BW and Ht were measured with subjects wearing light clothing without shoes. Body mass index (BMI) was calculated by dividing BW in kilograms by the square of height in meters (kg/m^2).

2.2 Dual energy X-ray absorptiometry (DXA)

The percentage of fat (% body fat) and bone mineral content (BMC) of the whole body and appendicular lean soft tissue (LST) were measured by DXA (Hologic QDR-4500 DXA Scanner and Hologic QDT DXA Scanner; Hologic Inc., Whaltham, MA, USA). Fat-free mass (FFM) and fat mass (FM) were calculated by BW and % body fat.

2.3 Method for the calculation of tissue organ mass

Tissue organ mass was calculated using the previously reported prediction model as follows. Bone mass (BM) was calculated by multiplying BMC times 1.85 (Snyder et al., 1975; Heymsfield et al., 1990). Adipose tissue mass (AT) was assumed to be 85% of total body fat (Heymsfield et al., 2002), leading to the model based on FM. Thus, AT was calculated by multiplying FM times 1.18. Skeletal muscle mass (SM) was calculated using the prediction model of Kim et al. (2002). Finally, residual mass (RM) was calculated as the difference between BW and the sum of the calculated BM, AT and SM. Residual mass includes all of the high-metabolic-rate tissues and organs such as heart, brain, liver, kidneys, spleen, and gastrointestinal tract.

$$\text{BM (kg)} = \text{BMC (g)} \times 1.85/1000$$
$$\text{AT (kg)} = \text{FM (kg)} \times 1.18$$
$$\text{SM (kg)} = 1.13 \times \text{LST (kg)} - 0.02 \times \text{age (years)} + 0.97$$
$$\text{RM (kg)} = \text{BW} - (\text{BM} + \text{AT} + \text{SM})$$

3. Resting energy expenditure (REE)

3.1 Method for measuring REE

Participants came to the laboratory either on the previous night and stayed overnight, or came in the morning. In the latter case, subjects were asked to minimize any walking while en route from their home to the laboratory before REE determination. The measured REE (REEm) was directly measured by open-circuit indirect calorimetry. Measurements were performed between 0700 and 0900 h after 10–12 h of fasting, except for water, in a room at constant room temperature (23–25℃). After entering the laboratory, subjects rested in the supine position for at least 30 min, and a face mask was put on. In the case of overnight stay, the subjects were quietly awakened at 0630 and were attached a face mask while remaining in bed for 30 minutes. Two samples of expired air were collected in Douglas bags for a duration of 10 min each, and the mean value was used for the analysis. For young subjects, all measurements were made during the follicular phase of the menstrual cycle. An oxygen and carbon dioxide analyzer (Arco-1000A; Arco system, Japan and AE-300; Minato Medical Science, Tokyo) was used to analyze the rate of oxygen consumption and carbon dioxide production. The volume of expired air was determined using a dry gas volume meter (DC-5; Shinagawa, Japan) and converted to standard temperature, standard pressure and dry gas. Gas exchange results were converted to REE (kcal/day) using Weir's equation (Weir, 1949). To examine whether overnight stay before the REE measurement caused a significant difference in the observed REE, analysis of covariance with REE as the dependent variable and age, height, FFM, and FM as covariates was employed. No significant effect of the measurement conditions was observed (overnight stay: 1169 ± 12 kcal/day (mean ± standard error (SE)), came in the early morning on the day: 1170 ± 7 kcal/day (mean ± SE), $F = 0.001$, $p = 0.980$).

3.2 Method for estimating REE

Estimation of REE using DXA was obtained based on the sum of four body compartments (BM, AT, SM and RM) times the corresponding tissue respiration rates as follows. The specific resting metabolic rate of the four compartments was assumed from previously reported data, bone (2.3 kcal/kg), AT (4.5 kcal/kg), skeletal muscle (13 kcal/kg) and residual (54 kcal/kg) (Holliday et al., 1967; Grande, 1989; Elia, 1992; Hayes et al., 2002; Heymsfield et al., 2002).

$$\text{REE (kcal/day)} = 2.3 \times BM + 4.5 \times AT + 13 \times SM + 54 \times RM$$

Predictive equations (kcal/day)	Age range	
DXA	-	2.3×BM + 4.5×AT + 13×SM + 54×RM
Harris-Benedict	-	655.0955 + 9.5634×BW + 1.8496×Ht - 4.6756×A
Schofield	18-29	(0.062×BW + 2.036)×1000/4.186
	30-59	(0.034×BW + 3.538)×1000/4.186
	60 over	(0.038×BW + 2.755)×1000/4.186
FAO/WHO/UNU	18-29	(55.6×BW + 1397.4×Ht/100 + 146)/4.186
	30-59	(36.4×BW - 104.6×Ht/100 + 3619)/4.186
	60 over	(38.5×BW + 2665.2×Ht/100 - 1264)/4.186
DRI (Japan)	18-29	22.1 ×BW
	30-49	21.7 ×BW
	50 over	20.7 ×BW
NIHN (Japan)	-	(0.0481×BW + 0.0234×Ht - 0.0138×A - 0.9708)×1000/4.186

BM: bone mass (kg), AT: adipose tissue mass (kg), SM: skeletal muscle mass (kg), RM: residual mass (kg), BW: body weight (kg), Ht: height (cm), A: age (years).

Table 1. Predictive equations of resting energy expenditure for women used in the present study.

3.3 Predictive equations of REE for women

Other predictive REEs were calculated using the Harris–Benedict (Harris & Benedict, 1919), Schofield (Schofield, 1985), FAO/WHO/UNU (FAO/WHO/UNU, 1985), DRI (Japan) (Ministry of Heaith, Labour and Welfare of Japan, 2009), and NIHN (Japan) (Ganpule et al., 2007) equations (Table 1).

4. The validity of body composition measurement using DXA for estimating REE

4.1 Subjects

The data used for the current analysis were collected from different 3 experimental studies that followed a similar methodology (Usui et al., 2009; Taguchi et al., 2011; Hasegawa et al., 2011). Total of 288 healthy women (216 young women; age: 21.8 ± 2.0 (18-29) years and 72 elderly women; age: 63.3 ± 6.4 (50-77) years) were recruited for the study. The elderly subjects had passed three years or more (13.5 ± 7.4 years) after menopause. None had used medications that affect bone and estrogen replacement was eliminated from the analysis. All subjects were informed about the purpose and possible risks of the study and were then provided written informed consent. These studies were conducted according to the guidelines laid down in the Declaration of Helsinki. All procedures involving human subjects were approved by the Ethical Committee of the National Institute of Health and Nutrition in Tokyo, the Institutional Ethical Committee Review Board of Japan Women's College of Physical Education in Tokyo, and the Human Research Ethical Committee of the Faculty of Sport Sciences of Waseda University, in Saitama.

4.2 Statistical analysis

Results are presented as the mean ± standard deviation (SD). Statistical analyses were carried out with the Sigma Stat 3.5 (Systat Software Inc., CA, USA). Statistical analysis was performed using the Student's t-test for parametric variables and the Mann-Whitney rank sum test for nonparametric variables to determine differences between young and elderly women. In addition to the mean ± SD of the difference, total error was used to determine how accurately predicted REE matched measured REE. This statistic includes two sources of variation, one attributable to the lack of association between the two sets of measurement (standard error of estimate) and one attributable to the difference between the means (van der Ploeg et al., 2001). Statistical significance of differences between measured and predicted values in all subjects was analyzed by one-way repeated-measures analysis of variance (ANOVA) and Dunnett's post hoc test. Evaluation of bias between measured and predicted REE was conducted with a Bland–Altman analysis (Bland and Altman, 1986). Fixed bias was indicated if the 95% coefficient interval (CI) for the difference between measured and predicted REE did not include zero. Predictive equations that are accurate display a tight prediction interval around zero. The 95%CI below zero signify an underestimation, while the 95%CI above zero signify an overestimation. The correlation of the difference between measured and predicted REE values and the mean from the both REE values was utilized to assess proportional bias. Statistical significance was set at $p < 0.05$ for all predictors.

4.3 Results

Table 2 presents the comparisons of subjects characteristics and body composition. Ht was significantly lower in the elderly women (50 over age group) than in young women (18-29 age group). However, no significant difference in BW was noted between two groups. The elderly women had significantly higher levels of % body fat and FM, and lower levels of FFM than the young group. When the FFM was separated into BM, SM, and RM, young women had significantly higher BM, SM, and RM than elderly women.

	All	Age range	
		18-29	50 over
	n = 288	n = 216	n = 72
Age (years)	32.1 ± 18.4	21.8 ± 2.0	63.3 ± 6.4 †
Ht (cm)	159.7 ± 6.8	161.6 ± 6.2	153.9 ± 5.2 *
BW (kg)	54.8 ± 7.4	54.9 ± 7.8	54.3 ± 6.0
BMI (kg/m^2)	21.5 ± 2.6	21.0 ± 2.5	22.9 ± 2.3 *
FFM (kg)	41.4 ± 5.8	42.6 ± 5.9	37.7 ± 3.5 †
FM (kg)	13.4 ± 4.0	12.3 ± 3.4	16.6 ± 3.9 †
% body fat	24.3 ± 5.8	22.3 ± 4.6	30.2 ± 4.8 *
BM (kg)	3.8 ± 0.7	4.0 ± 0.6	3.1 ± 0.5 †
AT (kg)	15.8 ± 4.7	14.5 ± 4.0	19.6 ± 4.6 †
SM (kg)	19.5 ± 3.5	20.5 ± 3.3	16.5 ± 1.9 †
RM (kg)	15.7 ± 2.1	15.9 ± 2.2	15.2 ± 1.5 †

Means ± SD, Ht: Height, BW: body weight, BMI: body mass index, FFM: fat-free mass, FM: fat mass, BM: bone mass, AT: adipose tissue mass, SM: skeletal muscle mass, RM: residual mass, * $p<0.05$ vs. 18-29 age group (Student's t-test), † $p<0.05$ vs. 18-29 age group (Mann-Whitney rank sum test).

Table 2. Physical characteristics in the healthy women.

Table 3 show measured and predicted REEs, and the mean and total errors of predicted REEs. No significant differences were observed from the REEm in predicted REE values by using DXA, DRI (Japan) equation, and NIHN (Japan) equation in all subjects. On the other hand, the mean errors of REE predicted by the Harris-Benedict, Schofield, and FAO/WHO/UNU equations were significantly higher than the REEm in all subjects. Total error of estimated REE by using DXA was lowest in the group. Total error using NIHN (Japan) equation was the second to the lowest. In particular, total error of the Harris-Benedict equation was largest in healthy women.

The systemic bias between the measured and predicted REEs by the Bland-Altman analysis are shown in Table 4 and Fig. 1. Fixed bias was not present in only estimated REE by using DXA. However, the REE estimated by using DXA had a proportional bias (Fig. 1 (a)). Systematic bias (fixed and proportional bias) was presented in predicted REE by the Harris-Benedict, Schofield, FAO/WHO/UNU, and NIHN (Japan) equations.

All subjects (n = 288)	REE (kcal/day)	Mean error[a] (kcal/day)		Total error[b] (kcal/day)
REEm (kcal/day)	**1170 ± 167**			
predicted REE				
DXA	**1181 ± 152**	**11 ± 104**		**105**
Harris-Benedict	**1324 ± 123**	**154 ± 121**	c	**196**
Schofield	**1273 ± 119**	**104 ± 111**	c	**151**
FAO/WHO/UNU	**1281 ± 118**	**111 ± 109**	c	**156**
DRI (Japan)	**1191 ± 166**	**22 ± 114**		**115**
NIHN (Japan)	**1184 ± 136**	**14 ± 110**		**111**

Means ± SD.; [a] Mean error = predicted REE – measured REE. ; [b] Total error (kcal/day) = $\sqrt{(\sum(\text{predicted REE} - \text{measured REE})^2/n)}$. ; [c] $p<0.05$ vs. measured REE (one-way repeated-measures ANOVA and Dunnett's post hoc test).

Table 3. Measured and predicted REE and cross-validation of REE prediction equations against the measured REE of healthy women.

	Bland-Altman analysis			
	fixed bias		proportional bias	
predicted REE	95%CI		r	*p* values
DXA	-1.1 ~ 23.0	N.S.	-0.152	p = 0.010
Harris-Benedict	140.2 ~ 168.3		-0.395	p < 0.001
Schofield	90.8 ~ 116.5		-0.471	p < 0.001
FAO/WHO/UNU	98.5 ~ 123.8		-0.481	p < 0.001
DRI (Japan)	8.4 ~ 34.8		-0.010	p = 0.868 N.S.
NIHN (Japan)	1.6 ~ 27.2		-0.307	p < 0.001

Table 4. Bland–Altman analysis.

4.4 Discussion

With the increasing availability of imaging methods, CT, MRI, and DXA, estimating methods of REE are developing and providing a "new" viewpoint of REE from the modeling perspective of organs and tissues. The importance of the developed approach is that it not only provides a qualitative estimate of REE, but of the actual distribution of heat-producing tissue components. As whole-body CT and MRI cannot assess body composition easily and quickly, previous investigators have explored the use of DXA as an available and practical alternative for developing qualitative tissue organ REE predictions. Hayes et al. (2002) demonstrated that REE can be estimated from five measured DXA values: body weight, total body fat mass, bone mineral content, appendicular lean mass, and head area. Their findings suggested that when REE is reviewed in the context of major heat-producing

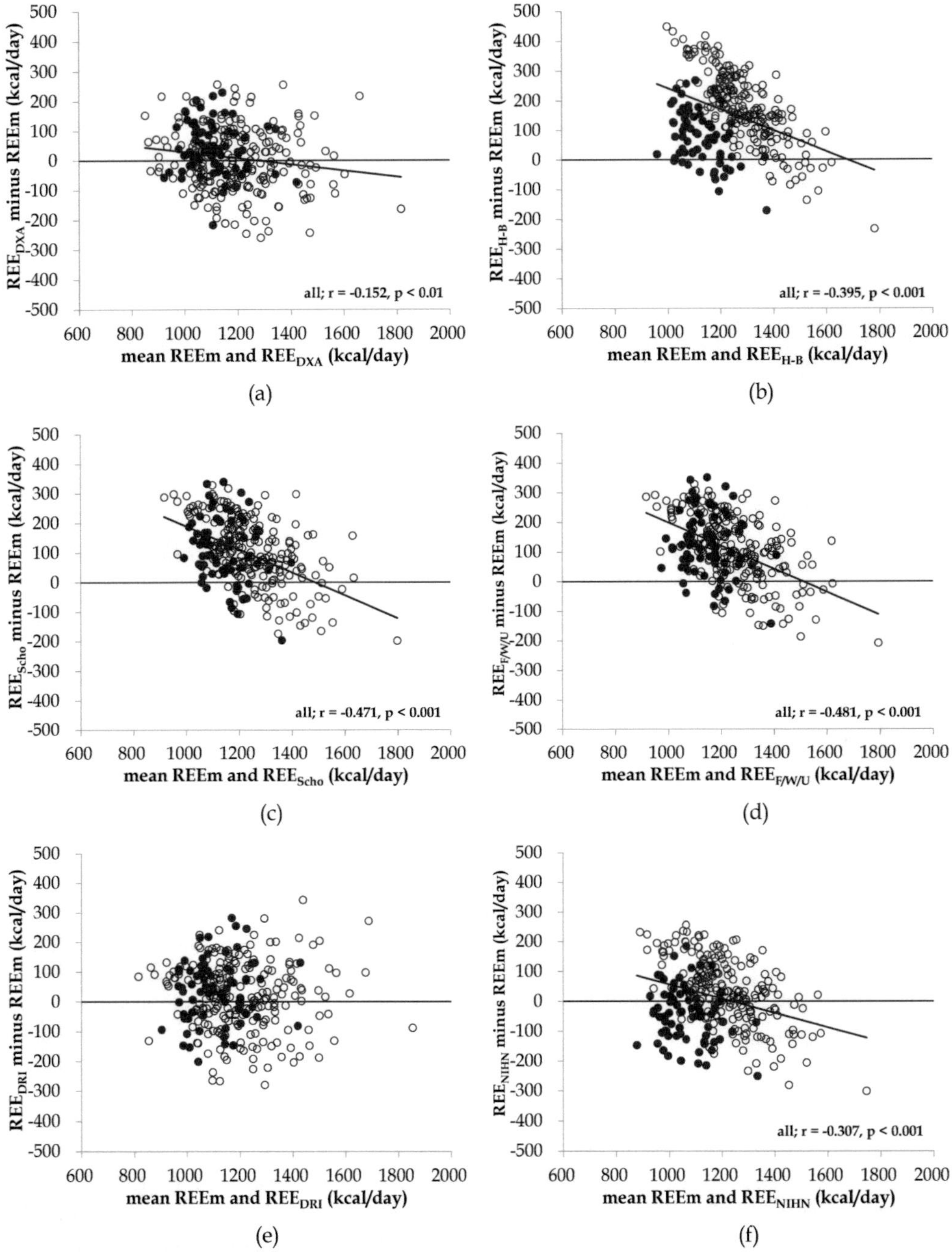

Plots of the differences between measured REE and predicted REE. Open circle (○): young subjects ($n = 216$), black circle (●): elderly subjects ($n = 72$), the solid line (-): regression line in all subjects ($n = 288$), REEm: measured by expiratory gas exchange, REE_{DXA}: estimated by using DXA, $REE_{H\text{-}B}$: predicted by Harris–Benedict equation, REE_{scho}: predicted by Schofield equations, $REE_{F/W/U}$: predicted by FAO/WHO/UNU equations, REE_{DRI}: predicted by DRI (Japan) equations, REE_{NIHN}: predicted by NIHN (Japan) equation.

Fig. 1. Bland–Altman plot.

units differing in metabolic activity, normal-weight men and women are actually quite similar. In addition, this five component model allowed REE prediction over a wide range of FFM, because the mean REE prediction errors in intermediate weight, underweight and obese subjects were not significantly different between groups (Bosy-Westphal et al., 2004). These findings provided indirect evidence for a view that, for practical purposes within humans, the specific metabolic rate is constant with increasing organ mass, and that interindividual REE differences in under- or overweight are more a reflection of an altered ratio of organ–tissue mass to body size.

On the other hand, there is evidence that REE is lower in the elderly, even after adjustment for tissue and organ mass (Gallagher et al., 2000) or age-related differences in body composition (Van Pelt et al., 1997, 2001). This raises the important question of the validity of assumed tissue- and organ-specific metabolic rates. The specific metabolic rates applied in the present study represent literature averages. The extent to which these heat production rates are valid remains unknown. Moreover, the specific metabolic rates for some components reported in the literature vary widely. However, we demonstrated that estimation based on the four tissue organs by using DXA allows successful calculation of REE in female adults regardless of age and aerobic fitness levels. (Usui et al., 2009). Our findings suggested the possibility that REE is regulated mainly by the mass of the tissue organs with lower and higher metabolic rates, including skeletal muscle and intestinal organs, rather than a decline in the specific metabolic rate of different tissue organs associated with advancing age and decreasing aerobic fitness levels in young and elderly women.

In addition, as for the four component model of REE prediction, Taguchi et al. (2011) evaluated that the relationship between REE and body composition in Japanese female athletes with a wide range of body sizes. Their results indicated, in good agreement with previous study (Bosy-Westphal et al., 2004), that REE for female athletes with a wide range of body sizes can be attributed to changes in organ tissue mass, and not changes in organ tissue metabolic rate. Moreover, Hasegawa et al. (2011) investigated the differences in body composition and REE between young women with low (BMI < 18.5 kg/m^2) and normal BMI ($18.5 \leqq$ BMI<25 kg/m^2), and suggested the possibility that low BMI subjects with normal menstrual cycle do not have any differences in specific metabolic rates of different tissue organs compared to those with normal BMI. According to Bland-Altman analysis in the present chapter, although there is a proportional bias in estimation of REE by using DXA, this proportional bias is relatively small compared with other estimation methods for REE (Table 4 and Fig. 1). Furthermore, fixed bias was not present in only estimated REE by using DXA. These findings suggested that estimation of the four tissue organs by using DXA can easily, practically, precisely, and accurately predict REE in healthy men and women.

The present chapter also focused on the validity of body composition measurement using DXA for estimating REE. Our results showed that predicted REE values by using DXA, DRI (Japan) equations, and NIHN (Japan) equation were not significantly different from the REEm, while Harris–Benedict, Schofield, and FAO/WHO/UNU equations significantly higher than the REEm in healthy women (Table 3). DRI (Japan) and NIHN (Japan) equations were developed based on the data for Japanese subjects with standard body size (Ministry of Heaith, Labour and Welfare of Japan, 2009; Ganpule et al., 2007). Schofield and FAO/WHO/UNU equations were developed based on data from a population of many races (Schofield, 1985; FAO/WHO/UNU, 1985). However, the data used to develop the Schofield equations were mostly from young European military and police recruits with 45% being of Italian descent. Harris–Benedict equation was developed using data obtained in healthy normal weight Caucasian men and women aged 15–74 years. Asians are reported to have lower REE than Europeans by 10–12% (Hayter et al., 1994), even after adjustment for body composition. According to a recent study by Miyake et al. (2011), mean difference and total error values were smaller using the DRI (Japan) equations and NIHN (Japan) equation than the internationally used equations (Harris–Benedict, Schofield, FAO/WHO/UNU) in both sexes. In particular, the total error was lower for the NIHN (Japan) equation than the other equations in most age groups (Miyake et al., 2011). In the present chapter, the mean errors of the predicted REEs by using DXA, DRI (Japan) equations, and NIHN (Japan) equation were smaller than those of internationally used equations in all subjects (Table 3). In addition, total error of estimated REE by using DXA, DRI (Japan) equations, and NIHN (Japan) equation were also lower than other total errors (105 kcal/day, 115 kcal/day, 111 kcal/day, respectively). Moreover, while these three prediction methods had some kind of bias, the bias was relatively small compared with other internationally used equations (Table 4 & Fig. 1 (a), (e), (f)). The results of this chapter supported the notions that the DRI (Japan) and NIHN (Japan) equations of REE are more accurate in healthy Japanese subjects, and that estimating REE from four tissue organ components by using DXA will be one of the useful methods for the dietary management (energetic assessment) in healthy Japanese subjects.

Our investigation has a few limitations. First, we did not test middle-aged (30–49 years) and very old (> 80 years) women and the adult men of all ages. It is unclear whether age-related functional decline in cells or tissue organs make a major impact on the heat production. Second, it was performed only in a Japanese population. Hayter et al. (1994) reported that Asians have lower REE than Europeans by 10–12%, even after adjustment for body composition. Third, because all the participants were healthy adult women, little is known as to whether this four component model for estimating REE by using DXA can accurately estimate REE in patients with a chronic disease, such as diabetes mellitus or cardiac disorder. Recently, DXA and regression modeling of REE showed that skeletal muscle is hypermetabolic in patients with HIV lipoatrophy (Kosmiski et al., 2009). Accordingly, the specific metabolic rate of each tissue organ may differ from those in healthy adults over 80 years of age, other ethnic subjects, or patients with a chronic disease. Future studies are needed to extend these observations and to analyze gender-related, genetics, hormonal, ethnic, and other determinant factors of REE.

5. Conclusion

The results of the present chapter suggest that REE in healthy adult women can be accurately estimated from four tissue organ components by using DXA, because the mean error, total error, and systematic bias between the predicted and measured REE was relatively small compared with other estimation methods for REE. Therefore, we expect that the DXA will be one of the useful methods not only for examining body composition and bone mineral density but also for estimating REE in a broad range of fields. In the future, DXA method may offer a bridge to effective prevention, treatment and care with the dietary management and exercise regimen for life style-related disease, such as obesity, osteoporosis, and type 2 diabetes.

6. Acknowledgments

We express our appreciation to the subjects for their cooperation in this study. We thank the members of the National Institute of Health and Nutrition and Waseda University for their help in this experiment. This study was supported by a Research Grant for Academic Frontier Projects from the Ministry of Education, Culture, Sports, Science and Technology (05F-02), a Waseda University Grant for Special Research Projects (2005A-932, 2006B-242), Health Sciences Research Grants from the Ministry of Health, Labor and Welfare, Medical Health Care Research Grants from the Consolidated Research Institute for Advanced Science and Medical Care at Waseda University, Research grant for Waseda University Global COE program: Sports Sciences for Promotion of Active Life (projectsIII-2), Research Grant from Japan Women's College of Physical Education, and Research Grants from the Japanese Olympic Committee.

7. References

Bland, J.M. & Altman, D.G. (1986). Statistical methods for assessing agreement between two methods of clinical measurement. *The Lancet*, Vol.327, No.8476, (08 February 1986), pp. 307–310, Print ISSN 0140-6736

Bosy-Westphal, A.; Reinecke, U.; Schlörke, T.; Illner, K.; Kutzner, D.; Heller M. & Müller, M.J. (2004). Effect of organ and tissue masses on resting energy expenditure in underweight, normal weight and obese adults. *International Journal of Obesity and Related Metabolic Disorders*, Vol.28, No.1, (January 2004), pp. 72–79, Print ISSN 0307-0565, Online ISSN 1476-5497

Elia, M. (1992). Organ and tissue contribution to metabolic rate. In: *Energy Metabolism: Tissue Determinants and Cellular Corollaries*, Kinney, J. M. & Tucker, H. N. (eds), pp. 61–80, Raven Press, ISBN 978-088-1678-71-0, New York

FAO/WHO/UNU. (1985). *Energy and protein requirements, report of a joint FAO/WHO/UNU expert consultation. Technical Report Series 724*, WHO, ISBN 92-4-120724-8, Geneva.

Fukagawa, N.K.; Bndini, L.G. & Young, J.B. (1990). Effect of age on body composition and resting metabolic rate. *American Journal of Physiology Endocrinology and Metabolism*, Vol.259, No.2, (August 1990), pp. E233–E238, Print ISSN 0193-1849, Online ISSN 1522-1555

Gallagher, D.; Belmonte, D.; Deurenberg, P.; Wang, Z.; Krasnow, N.; Pi-Sunyer, F.X. & Heymsfield S.B. (1998). Organ-tissue mass measurement allows modeling of REE and metabolically active tissue mass. *American Journal of Physiology Endocrinology and Metabolism*, Vol.275, No.2, (August 1998), pp. E249–E258, Print ISSN 0193-1849, Online ISSN 1522-1555

Gallagher, D.; Allen, A.; Wang, Z.; Heymsfield, S.B. & Krasnow, N. (2000). Smaller organ tissue mass in the elderly fails to explain lower resting metabolic rate. *Annals of the New York Academy of Sciences*, Vol.904, (May 2000), pp. 449–455, Print ISSN 0077-8923, Online ISSN 1749-6632

Ganpule, A.A.; Tanaka, S.; Ishikawa-Takata, K. & Tabata, I. (2007). Interindividual variability in sleeping metabolic rate in Japanese subjects. *European Journal of Clinical Nutrition*, Vol.61, No.11, (Epub February 2007), pp. 1256–1261, Print ISSN 0954-3007, Online ISSN 1476-5640

Grande, F. (1980). Energy expenditure of organs and tissues. In: *Assessment of Energy Metabolism in Health and Disease: Report of the First Ross Conference on Medical Research*, Kinney, J.M. (ed.), pp. 88–92, Ross Laboratories, Columbus, Ohio

Harris, J.A. & Benedict, F.G. (1919). *A Biometric Study of Basal Metabolism in Man*, Washington, Publication, No. 279, Carnegie Institute of Washington, ISBN 978-114-4176-76-9, Washington D.C.

Hasegawa, A.; Usui, C.; Kawano, H.; Sakamoto, S. & Higuchi, M. (2011). Characteristics of body composition and resting energy expenditure in lean young women. *Journal of Nutritional Science and Vitaminology*, Vol.57, No.1, (January 2011), pp. 74-79, Print ISSN 0301-4800, Online ISSN 1881-7742

Hayes, M.; Chustek, M.; Wang, Z.; Gallagher, D.; Heshka, S.; Spungen, A.; Bauman, W. & Heymsfield S.B. (2002). DXA: potential for creating a metabolic map of organ-tissue resting energy expenditure components. *Obesity Research*, Vol.10, No.10, (October 2002), pp. 969–977, ISSN 1930-7381, Online ISSN 1930-739x

Hayter, J.E. & Henry, C.J.K. (1994). A re–examination of basal metabolic rate predictive equations: the importance of geographic origin of subjects in sample selection. *European Journal of Clinical Nutrition*, Vol.48, No.10, (October 1994), pp. 702-707, Print ISSN 0954-3007, Online ISSN 1476-5640

Heymsfield, S.B.; Smith, R.; Aulet, M.; Bensen, B.; Lichtman, S.; Wang, J. & Pierson, RN. (1990). Appendicular skeletal muscle mass: measurement by dualphoton absorptiometry. *American Journal of Clinical Nutrition*, Vol.52, No.2, (August 1990), pp. 214–218, Print ISSN 0002-9165, Online ISSN 1938-3207

Heymsfield, S.B.; Gallagher, D.; Kotler, D.P.; Wang, Z.; Allison, D.B. & Heshka, S. (2002). Body-size dependence of resting energy expenditure can be attributed to non-energetic homogeneity of fat-free mass. *American Journal of Physiology Endocrinology and Metabolism*, Vol.282, No.1, (January 2002), pp. E132–E138, Print ISSN 0193-1849, Online ISSN 1522-1555

Holliday, M.A.; Potter, D.; Jarrah, A. & Bearg, S. (1967). The relation of metabolic rate to body weight and organ size. *Pediatric Research*, Vol.1, No.3, (May 1967), pp. 185–195, Print ISSN 0031-3998, Online ISSN 1530-0447

Hunter, G.R.; Weinsier, R.L.; Gower, B.A. & Wetzstein, C. (2001). Age-related decrease in resting energy expenditure in sedentary white women: effects of regional differences in lean and fat mass. *American Journal of Clinical Nutrition*, Vol.73, No.2, (February 2001), pp. 333–337, Print ISSN 0002-9165, Online ISSN 1938-3207

Kim, J.; Wang, Z.; Heymsfield, S.B.; Baumgartner, R.N. & Gallagher, D. (2002). Total-body skeletal muscle mass: estimation by a new dual-energy X-ray absorptiometry method. *American Journal of Clinical Nutrition*, Vol.76, No.2, (August 2002), pp. 378–383, Print ISSN 0002-9165, Online ISSN 1938-3207

Kosmiski, L.A.; Ringham, B.M.; Grunwald, G.K. & Bessesen, D.H. (2009). Dual-energy X-ray absorptiometry modeling to explain the increased resting energy expenditure associated with the HIV lipoatrophy syndrome. *American Journal of Clinical Nutrition*, Vol.90, No.6, (December 2009), pp. 1525–1531, Print ISSN 0002-9165, Online ISSN 1938-3207

Mazes, R.B.; Barden, H.S.; Bisek, J.P. & Hanson J. (1990). Dual energy x-ray absorptiometry for total-body and regional bone-mineral and soft-tissue composition. *American*

Journal of Clinical Nutrition, Vol.51, No.6, (June 1990), pp. 1106–1112, Print ISSN 0002-9165, Online ISSN 1938-3207

Ministry of Heaith, Labour and Welfare of Japan. (2009). *Dietary reference intakes for Japanese, 2010*, Daiichi Shuppan, ISBN 978-4-8041-1219-0, Tokyo. (in Japanese)

Miyake, R.; Tanaka, S.; Ohkawara, K.; Ishikawa-Takata, K., Hikihara Y.; Taguri, E.; Kayashita J. & Tabata, I. (2011). Validity of predictive equations for basal metabolic rate in Japanese adults. *Journal of Nutritional Science and Vitaminology*, Vol.57, No.3 , (June 2011), pp. 224-232, Print ISSN 0301-4800, Online ISSN 1881-7742

Ravussin, E. & Bogardus, C. (1989). Relationship of genetics, age, and physical fitness to daily energy expenditure and fuel utilization. *American Journal of Clinical Nutrition*, Vol.49, No.5 supplements, (May 1989), pp. S968–S975, Print ISSN 0002-9165, Online ISSN 1938-3207

Schofield, W.N. (1985). Predicting basal metabolic rate, new standards and review of previous work. *Human Nutrition. Clinical Nutrition*, Vol.39, supplements, (1985), pp. 5–41, ISSN 0263-8290

Snyder, W.S.; Cook, M.J.; Nasset, E.S.; Karhausen, L.R.; Howells, G.P. & Tipton, I.H. (1975). *Report of the Task Group of Reference Man*, Pergamon Press, ISBN 00-8-017024-2, Oxford.

Svendsen, O.L.; Haarbo, J.; Heitman, B.L.; Gotfredsen, A. & Christiansen, C. (1991). Measurement of body fat in elderly subjects by dual energy x-ray absorptiometry, bioelectrical impedance, and anthropometry. *American Journal of Clinical Nutrition*, Vol.53, No.5, (May 1991), pp. 1117–1123, Print ISSN 0002-9165, Online ISSN 1938-3207

Svendsen, O.L.; Haarbo, J.; Hassager, C. & Christiansen, C. (1993). Accuracy of measurements of body composition by dual energy x-ray absorptiometry in vivo. *American Journal of Clinical Nutrition*, Vol.57, No.5, (May 1993), pp. 605–608, Print ISSN 0002-9165, Online ISSN 1938-3207

Taguchi, M.; Ishikawa-Takata, K.; Tatsuta, W.; Katsuragi, C.; Usui, C.; Sakamoto, S. & Higuchi M. (2011). Resting energy expenditure can be assessed by fat-free mass in female athletes regardless of body size. *Journal of Nutritional Science and Vitaminology*, Vol.57, No.1, (January 2011), pp. 22-29, Print ISSN 0301-4800, Online ISSN 1881-7742

Tataranni, P.A. & Ravussin, E. (1995). Variability in metabolic rate: biological sites of regulation. *International Journal of Obesity and Related Metabolic Disorders*, Vol.19, No.4 supplements, (October 1995), pp. S102–S106, Print ISSN 0307-0565, Online ISSN 1476-5497

Usui, C.; Takahashi, E.; Gando, Y.; Sanada, K.; Oka, J.; Miyachi, M.; Tabata, I. & Higuchi, M. (2009). Resting energy expenditure can be assessed by dual-energy X-ray absorptiometry in women regardless of age and fitness. *European Journal of Clinical Nutrition*, Vol.63, No.4, (Epub February 2008), pp. 529-535, Print ISSN 0954-3007, Online ISSN 1476-5640

van der Ploeg, G.E.; Gunn, S.M.; Withers, R.T.; Modra, A.C.; Keeves, J.P. & Chatterton, B.E. (2001). Predicting the resting metabolic rate of young Australian males. *European Journal of Clinical Nutrition*, Vol.55, No. 3, (March 2001), pp. 145–152, Print ISSN 0954-3007, Online ISSN 1476-5640

Van Pelt, R.E.; Dinneno, F.A.; Seals, D.R. & Jones, P.P. (2001). Age-related decline in RMR in physically active men: relation to exercise volume and energy intake. *American Journal of Physiology Endocrinology and Metabolism*, Vol.281, No.3, (September 2001), pp. E633–E639, Print ISSN 0193-1849, Online ISSN 1522-1555

Van Pelt, R.E.; Jones, P.P.; Davy, K.P.; Desouza, C.A.; Tanaka, H.; Davy, B.M. & Seals D.R. (1997). Regular exercise and the age-related decline in resting metabolic rate in women. *The Journal of Clinical Endocrinology and Metabolism*, Vol.82, No.10, (October 1997), pp. 3208–3212, Print ISSN 0021-972x, Online ISSN 1945-7197

Wang, Z.; Heshka, S.; Gallagher, D.; Boozer, C.N.; Kotler, D.P. & Heymsfield, S.B. (2000). Resting energy expenditure fat-free mass relationship: new insights provided by body composition modeling. *American Journal of Physiology Endocrinology and Metabolism*, Vol.279, No.3, (September 2000), pp. E539–E545, Print ISSN 0193-1849, Online ISSN 1522-1555

Weir, J.B. (1949). New methods for calculating metabolic rate with special reference to protein metabolism. *Journal of Physiology*, Vol.109, No.1-2, (August 1949), pp. 1-9, Print ISSN 0022-3751, Online ISSN 1469-7793

5

Dxa as a Tool for the Assessment of Morphological Asymmetry in Athletes

Magdalena Krzykała
University School of Physical Education in Poznań
Anthropology and Biometry Department,
Poland

1. Introduction

Symmetry and asymmetry - two opposite phenomenon, does coexist in nature and both are very essential for science. There are many definition of symmetry, depending on research area. In biology, a dominant view is the left-right bilateral symmetry describes health and high genetic quality (Gould & Gould, 1989). In physics, symmetry includes all features of a physical system that exhibit the property of symmetry—that is, under certain transformations, aspects of these systems are "unchanged according to a particular observation" (en.wikipedia.org). In mathematics, the intellectual pursuit of the Universal formulation of symmetry (Group Theory) has led to major discoveries in physics, and to Einstein's general relativity theory (Engler, 2005). In chemistry, left-right balance is a critical component in the notion of symmetry and refers to regular arrangements of molecules and the more symmetrical, the more aesthetic (Muller, 2003). Additionally symmetry and chemistry have been in interplay in spectroscopy, crystallography, reactivity and conformational analysis. Besides, symmetry considerations continua to assist chemistry in systematizing and interpreting observation and in discovering new reactions, molecules, and other material (Hargittai & Hargittai, 2005). In art, symmetry refers to left-right, top-bottom balance (of forms, colors, lines etc) in the composition as a whole being essential component of art's aesthetic quality (Jacobsen et al, 2006).

On the one hand symmetry means proper proportions, harmony, and balance between two elements of some totality and is connected with beauty. On the other hand there is another definition of this term- bilateral symmetry (right-left symmetry). Both of them concern body build (morphological symmetry), but can also refer to some human movements (Starosta, 1990).

According to Frey (1949) "symmetry signifies rest and binding, asymmetry motion and loosening, the one order and law, the other arbitrariness and accident, the one formal rigidity and constrains, the other life, play and freedom".

According to Webster dictionary (Webster, 1991) symmetry is quality of possessing exactly corresponding parts on either side of an axis and in biology - regularity in form or similarity of structure, whereas asymmetry it is lack of symmetry, uneven disposition on each side of an central line or point.

The opposite word to symmetry is asymmetry. Three kinds of asymmetry were distinguished by Wolański (1955): 1/ morphological - differences in size and shape of organs or body parts situated on left or right side of the body; 2/ functional - connected with one of hemispheres domination (usually left); 3/ dynamic - differences between left and right extremities in strength, muscles hardness and elasticity.

Bilateral asymmetry in humans, as was stated by same authors (Zeidel & Hessamian, 2010), was fashioned by millions of years of adaptive evolution and it implies perfection.

There are three types of bilateral asymmetry by Van Valen (1962): 1/directional asymmetry (DA): when some traits develop more on one side than the other, e.g., the human brain; 2/ antisymmetry: asymmetric development is typical, but unpredictable, e.g., larger signaling claw of the male fiddler crabs or handedness in human; 3/ fluctuating asymmetry (FA): "randomly produced deviations from perfect symmetry of two sides of quantitative traits in an individual for which the population mean of R-L differences is zero and their variability is near-normally distributed".

Normal human body asymmetry appear very soon and the manifestation of morphological asymmetry intensify with aging what is connected with functional asymmetry (Malinowski, 2004). Level of asymmetry among population reflects its developmental stability, hence differences between right and left bilateral trait are very good predictor of developmental stability both on the individually and population level. Fluctuating asymmetry has been the most widely used measure of developmental stability (Palmer & Strobeck, 1992).

Potentially human body is divided into two symmetrical parts but in fact there are some deviations (aberrations): 1) internal aberrations: asymmetry of even (kidney) and odd (pancreas, heart, spleen, liver, stomach etc) of internal organs. It refers to size, shape, location, constitution or function, 2) external aberration: refer to extremities asymmetry and handedness. There is strict connection of those aberrations with hemisphere domination (Czachowska-Sieszycka, 1983). The more increasing of the left hemisphere in domination, the more differences in left and right size of the brain. The fact that human brain is asymmetrically organized is known for about 140 years. Platon stated that symmetry is ideal (beauty is symmetrical and proportional) and that there are perfect harmony between one side to the other. That is why anthropologists in XIX w thought that human brain must be symmetrical. Paul Broca debunked this theory (Broca, 1865) and stated that right hemisphere damaged cripple speech rarely but left hemisphere - in most cases. On the basis of this information he found out that speech centers are localized only on the one side of the brain. Nowadays, the research including asymmetry of human brain are more and more advanced due to a new technology. It is valid, because the information about right and left hemisphere asymmetry could also help in better understanding of human body morphological diversification.

2. Morphological asymmetry in sport

In sport there is a need to seek some acts to achievements the highest results, especially in highest level athletes. Among other factors like training methods modification or biological regeneration also certain level of morphological parameters is very important. Body compartments, among other factors, play an important role in physical performance (Petersen et al., 2006). Generally, the body composition of athletes are consider in terms of whole body composition, but research show that regional BMD, FFM and FM distribution is equally important, in relation to training and performance (Bell et al., 2005). Tend to this direction more and more scientists conduct research in this area.

Many researches proved that morphological asymmetry - the difference between the right and the left sides of the body exist in sport (Dorado et al., 2002; Auerbach & Ruff 2006; Starosta, 1990) and it is very important to observe the scale of this phenomenon in order to its elimination if it will be necessary. Morphological asymmetry can concerns both side-to-side differences between extremities, pelvis, trunk and total body with upper and lower body diversification. Analysis concerns mostly body dimension (length of limbs), level of body fat, lean and body density. In humans, some level of asymmetry in body dimensions is rather norm than the exception (Al-Eisa et al., 2004). It is stated that the lifelong preference for one extremity -e.g. the left arm or the left leg -as well as a predilection for a certain direction when turning around or rotating about one's longitudinal axis could lead to asymmetry which occurred in morphological characteristics and which can even be osseous in the case of competitive athletes. The body response on training stimulus will be vary according to its timing, duration and intensity (Malina, 1979).

It is obvious that morphological side–to–side diversification depends on sport specificity. Participation in asymmetric sport disciplines is connected with asymmetric changes in soft tissues (Ducher et al., 2005; Haapasalo et al., 1998). As was noticed, soft tissues indicate greater lateral differences than skeletal measurements (Van Dusen, 1939; Chhibber & Singh, 1970; Kimura & Asaeda, 1974;). Observation from literature suggests that in most cases the upper limb is laterally dominant in size on the right side while the lower limb is larger on the left side (Singh, 1970; McGrew & Marchant, 1997). Some studies stated that asymmetries are more pronounced in the upper extremities in comparison to lower extremities when the right side tends to be larger than the left (Munter, 1936; Tomkinson et al., 2003; Malina & Buschang, 2004; Ulijaszek & Mascie-Taylor, 2005). Malinowski (2004) stated that average, the right arm and forearm are longer, and larger are their circumferences. Left hand is longer and narrowest. The right upper limb is longer about 1 cm in comparison to left one, whereas left lower limb is longer about 10-13 mm. Also left foot, left thigh and calf circumferences are longer.

As was stated by some authors (Manning et al., 2002) small percentage changes in left or right trait size may result in large percentage changes in asymmetries, so precise and the most suitable method is need to evaluated regional morphological diversification among very specific part of population – athletes.

2.1 Methods for regional body composition assessment

There are different methods which could be use to do such analysis, which differ in the time, expense and accuracy of the results. These procedures are subject to some error which can result from measurement procedures, from the equations selected to calculate body fat percent, or from both. A standard error for most procedure is about 3 to 4 %.

The most traditional method to assess the size of particularly body segments is anthropometry. It uses circumferences, SKF thicknesses, skeletal breadth and segment lengths for total and regional body composition evaluation (Heyward & Wagner, 2004). Some standardized procedures should be taken into consideration to increase the accuracy and reliability of measurements like taking three measurements within ± 0.2 for body segments with relatively small girths (calf, arm, forearm) and three measurements within ± 1.0 cm for longer body segments like waist, abdomen and buttock; or using a small sliding caliper with greater precision to measure breadth of smaller segments (elbow, wrist) and so on (Wilmore et al., 1988). Schell and co-authors (Schell et al., 1985) emphasized that asymmetry of paired dimensions is a big methodological problem in anthropometry. Additionally, analysis of asymmetry should be done with advanced statistical tests. Moreover, interpretation of given results must be done with cautions especially, if observed differences are so small that could be lower than technical errors of measurement (Moreno et al., 2002).

There are also some newer methods to assess regional diversification of some tissues. Traditional BIA method, allows to assess only whole body composition (wrist-to-ankle), however segmental BIA (SBIA) system based on eight symmetrically re-positioned electrodes can give information about resistance and reactance values from right and left arms and legs and torso (www.rjlsystem.com/pdf-files/segmental_bia.pdf). Because of human body segments are not uniform in length or cross-sectional area, there will be different resistance to the flow of current through them (Heyward & Wagner., 2004). Fuller and Elia (1989) stated that those body segments which have small cross-sectional areas have simultaneously the greatest effect on impedance. The resistance ratio of upper limb-trunk-lower limb theoretically equal 13.8 : 1 : 11.8. SBIA measuring particularly body segments like upper and lower limb or trunk may be a good method for person with altered fluid distribution, so also for athletes (Organ et al., 1994). Segmental muscle changes for example during physical activity are visible by studying the individual arms and legs as a comparative percentage or a percent change over time. Segmental measurements can be successful made by traditional electrodes Akern Sre (Florence, Italy) or by segmental body composition analyzers (Omron, Tanita, BioSpace) which incorporate foot and hand contact points (where standing person holding two rods with fingers and thumb of each hand) what has disadvantage: high resistance of the body ankle and wrist are included in the measurements. Additionally the ankle, wrist, lower leg and forearm contribute more than 50 percent of the measurement (Scheltinge et al., 1991).

MRI (Magnetic Resonans Imaging) – another method to assess regional diversification, can be used to assess whole mass and muscle content of any body area, giving high-quality images of different tissues (Malina et al., 2004). Also computerized tomography CT is often used in regional determination of body segments with body fat, muscle and bone area assessment (Buckley et al., 1987; Forbes et al., 1988; Jordao et al., 2004). Magnetic resonance imaging and computed tomography are regard as the reference methods for regional body composition assessment but routine use of them is impeded by access, high cost, and in case of CT, significant exposure to ionizing radiation. Some authors propose then DXA (Dual Energy X-ray absorptiometry) as a more valid and precise method for measuring total and regional body composition (Chen et al., 2007; Andreoli et al., 2009). Generally, DXA, CT and MRI methods are consider to be a standard for precision and accuracy for body composition measurements (Chettle & Fremlin, 1984; Ellis, 2000). DXA is primary method to estimate body composition of the total body and specific regions (bone mineral, fat-free soft tissue and fat). The main assumption of absorptiometry method relies on measuring attenuation of X-rays with high-and-low-photon energies what is dependent on the thickness, density and chemical composition of the underlying tissue (Pietrobelli et al., 1996). Two kinds of absorptiometry were distinguished: single-photon absorptiometry and dual-photon absorptiometry which were precisely described in Lukaski comprehensive study (1987). It was stated that both technologies provide highly reproducible estimates of lean tissue mainly in adults, because the coefficient of variation for them for repeated measurements is less than 2 %. The advantage of DXA technology is reduced of radiation exposure and more readily available data about changes in bone mineral content in whole and regional skeleton. As was stated by Webber (1995) the x-ray exposure is low and corresponding to natural radiation and radioactivity received during 5 days of normal living. Additionally, this method is more relevant in longitudinal study to track changes in body composition (Malina et al., 2004) because of the good precision of particular DXA device (about 1% for BMC and 2-3% for total body fat) for assessing whole body composition (De Lorenzo et al., 1998).

Kistrop with co-authors (Kistrop et al., 2000) found that measuring total and regional body composition by DXA can improve the prediction of energy expenditure what could be a valid information for athletes who try to lose fat mass or gain lean muscle.

Each method has its own advantages and disadvantages, also DXA. Some authors observed (Calbet et al., 1998) that this method giving a general idea about the specific sport loading influence on BMC. On the other hand it is not possible to assess the effect of sport participation to particular bones during DXA analysis because it includes all bone structures. There are also some concerns about measurements bias related to the impact of a significant change in the lean tissue hydration. Some study however show not significantly alters the estimates for the bone, lean and fat mass (Pietrobelli et al., 1998). Another problem is that thicknesses are different depends on body regions and individual body shapes, so there could be large variation in percent fat in DXA study (Steward & Hannan, 2000b; Lohman & Chen, 2005). When comparing results of regional body composition from DXA scanners of different manufacturers, caution must be done because of some factors which are different among both of them like: pixel size, X-ray voltages or algorithms for shape and edge detection (Tothill et al., 1994; Steward & Hannan, 2000a). As was stated by some authors (Lohman & Chen, 2005) differences between DXA instruments from leading manufactures like Hologic, Lunar and Norland were 7% for body fat and about 15% for bone mineral content, some times ago. Nowadays, DXA software are more and more accurate with new calibration modes increasing precision and accuracy (O'Connor, 2006). iDXA (Lunar) for example have a little bit precision with total-body assessment and almost identical values in regional BMD measurements in comparison to Lunar Prodigy (Faulkner, 2006). Despite all limitations DXA is a widely used method, owing to its ease of use, availability, low-radiation exposure, good accuracy and reproducibility for the assessment of regional body composition. It is also seems to be less dependent on biological consistency than other methods (Haarbo et al., 1991; Kohrt, 1995) and is most useful for research purposes (Speiser et al., 2005). It was documented that regional adiposity by DXA is potentially more accurate than anthropometry measures, and more practical than computed tomography or magnetic resonance imaging scans (Henche et al., 2008). Taking into account all of those data, DXA seems to be one of the most suitable method for evaluation side-to-side morphological diversification among athletes.

2.2 Morphological asymmetry of athletes - research overview

Many studies with athletes body asymmetry exploited anthropometric method. Malina and Buschang (2004) observed greater hypertrophy in the musculature of the dominant side in athletes. Also another authors (Calbet et al., 2001; Dorado et al., 2002) found, on the example of golfers, that they had muscle hypertrophy in the dominant compared with non-dominant arm under training influence. The right-left differences in morphological parameters (mainly in forearm girth, arm girth, elbow width) were observed also in 134 athletes aged 21-32 years, engaged in many different asymmetric movement sports like tennis, canoeing, kayaking and boxing (Krawczyk et al., 1998). According to those research, most significant asymmetry was found among tennis players, then in kayakers, canoeists, rowers and skaters and concerned mainly forearm girth. The extreme directional asymmetry in the use of the limbs among tennis players is connected with physiological and anatomical changes in those body segments (Lucki, 2006). On the basis of 25 male collegiate tennis players age 19-24 from four NCAA Division I she stated that there was significant asymmetry between the limbs, related to cross-sectional measurements (circumferences, widths). Some authors (Maughan et al., 1986) observed greater proportion of muscle and smaller proportion of fat in dominant arm than the opposite limb in tennis players. Numerous studies indicated increased bone density in the dominant limb among tennis players (Ruff et al., 1994; Ducher et al., 2005; Lucki & Nicolay, 2007). Analysis of the bilateral asymmetry among collegiate (19-24 years old) tennis players showed that forearm circumferences of the dominant limb was greater than in the opposite limb (3-10% in female and 2-13% in male tennis players) (Lucki & Nikolay, 2007). Jone's (Jones et al., 1977) study examining site-specific accretion of bone of professional tennis players, with differences being up to 30%. Tarociński (1977) stated that difference in circumferences of the left and the right upper extremities was 1-2 cm in male athlete (age 12-15) playing tennis for four years, whereas in Marchwicki study (1927) those differences was smaller and equal 0,3 - 1,1 cm. also among young tennis players. In lower extremities, in turn, there was smaller diversification with left leg advantage (Tarociński, 1977). Similar finding was done later on the example of baseball players (Komi 1996; Bubanj & Obradovic, 2002).

Abraho and Mello (2008) made comparison of the young athletes playing tennis for at most two years (age 6-10 years) with the male instructors between 22 y and 37 years of age engaged in this sport discipline at least eight years. They noticed the increase of the incidence of right somatic measures superior to the left, because the excessive time of training of asymmetric sport. This situation has influence on postural deviation according to those research.

When one considers that carrying loads with the preferred hand means a stress on the arm muscles of the same side and a simultaneous activation of the contra-lateral muscles for the stabilization of one's balance, these functional asymmetries become plausible. It is also remarkable that hurdlers, high jumpers and pole vaulters exhibit higher muscle contractility in their swing leg than in their take-off leg (Absauomov, 1976) because of the higher mechanical load. Kruger et al (2005) determined the degree of upper body morphological asymmetry in 19 elite international male javelin throwers, age of 26,4 ± 4.4 years. They found larger variables on the dominant side for thirteen of the fourteen variables (especially for triceps skinfold 5.9%, half-chest girth 4.9%,, forearm girth 3.9%, biceps skinfold 2.5%) what could have health consequences and performance limiting effects. The morphological asymmetry in the upper body of fast bowlers in cricket was observed in Grobbelaar study (Grobbelaar et al., 2000). It concerns the relaxed arm (3.8 %), tensed arm (4.7%), forearm (2.8%) and ½ chest circumferences (6.4%).

The morphological characteristics of fencers show a typical asymmetry of the limbs as a result of the asymmetrical sport activity practicing what is advantage in gaining success. Fencing produces typical functional asymmetries that emphasize the very high level of specific function, strength and control required in this sport discipline (Roi et al., 2008). Muscle mass of dominant lower limb of high-class fencer is bigger than contrlateral limb (Nystrom et al., 1990). Tsolakis et al (2006) stated, on the example of fencers, that there was difference in morphological asymmetry of arm and leg depended on age, where arm asymmetries were specific for the age of 10-13 years, whereas leg asymmetries were observed among 14-17 year-old athletes. Because of asymmetrical nature of this sport, some specific injuries are characteristics in the shoulders, the back and the pelvic girdle, so there is necessity of including prevention in daily fencers training (Kucera & Henn, 2003).

Manning and Pickup (Manning, & Pickup, 1998) stated that the national league athletes would be more symmetric, because symmetry is positively related with physical performance in adult males. Besides, symmetric males run faster than asymmetric males (Manning & Pickup, 1998). According to Chinn study "Morphological asymmetry is more pointed out in high level athlete in case of asymmetrical sport disciplines" (Chinn et al., 1974). Tomkinson et al stated (2003) that there are no differences in variance in fluctuating asymmetry between adult basketball and soccer, competing at two different standards (professional national league and semi-professional state league).

There is also some assumption that symmetry positive correlated with body size what mean that the larger men is (higher and heavier), the more symmetric he is. But in women body size correlated negatively with symmetry (Manning, 1995). Additionally this author observed positive correlation between body mass index (BMI) and asymmetry among women (the bigger BMI= the bigger asymmetry). On the other hand some research indicated that the bigger person (both men and women)- the greater asymmetry (Graham et al., 1998).

Studies of scientists from many disciplines suggest that age, sex and environmental stress like extreme unilateral work are the most influential factors for morphological asymmetry (Wolański, 1962; Singh, 1970; Mascie-Taylor et al., 1981; Malina, 1983). Some authors also found (Hetland et al., 1998) that there are different factors significantly contributed to the regional body composition. On the basic of 108 (86 recreational and 22 elite runners) male long-distance runners they stated that training was the strongest determinant in the legs and the arms, whereas androgenic activity was important in the abdominal region. Some data suggest that persistent unilateral training may also influence specific bone lengths and width. As was stated by Buskirk et al (1956) on the example of seven tennis players (nationally level), the athletes had greater length and width of bones of the dominant hands and forearms than the non-dominant extremity. Authors suggested that those laterality differences were results of vigorous exercise on the bone growth during the adolescent years. Similar findings were done by Prives (1969).

In Jones et al study (1977) there was a significant hypertrophy of cortical bone of the humerus in the dominant arm compared to the non-playing arm of 84 male professional tennis players. There were sex differences in cortical thickness of the dominant arm compared to non-dominant arm among athletes (man had 35% greater cortical thickness of the dominant arm, whereas women - 28%). Hypertrophy of the humeral cortex has been reported also in the throwing arms of professional baseball pitchers (King et al., 1969).

Asymmetry could have different value and it is stated that when it access some level, it may hinder some special activity practice, could negatively affect the health (being connected with functional asymmetry and some changes for example in the area of backbone). According to Wilk et al study (2002) therapist should focus on restoring the functional shoulder asymmetry during rehabilitation of shoulder injuries in the case of throwing athlete. Asymmetries between lower limbs during athletic movements are thought to increase the risk of injury and compromise performance (Cronin, 2010). In the case of athletes who are engaged with sport discipline including one-sided hips rotation (tennis, golf, squash) and suffer from LBP, more lower limbs asymmetry and pelvic asymmetry (LLD-leg length discrepancy) were observed (Egan et al., 1995; Van Dillen et al., 2008). Some authors asked the question if the asymmetry lead to the back pain or did the back pain lead to the asymmetry (Bussey, 2010). This is not yet determined evolutionary dilemma. She stated that asymmetries may be functional adaptations, meaning that the body has successfully adapted to the asymmetrical loading demands of the sport in order to decrease the excessive strain in some tissues. Similar finding did previously Koszczyc (1991) who observed that shoulder and whole upper limb asymmetry (which can appear in progressive stadium of ontogeny) could be effect of body adaptation to increased mechanical loads. Bussey (2010) conducted the study based on 60 women divided into three groups consisted of elite athletes at the national and international level (bilateral group: triathlon, cross-country running, single scull rowing ; unilateral group: field hockey, ice hockey, speed-skating) and control group. She speculated that some level of pelvis asymmetry may be a natural effect of lateral dominance which decrease with bilateral activities like running or cycling or increase with unilateral nature of sport discipline like hockey.

Field hockey is one-side dominant sport. It means that athletes have preference of one side of the body over the other. There are many different specific movements in this discipline. Many of them involve a rapid rotation of the hips, shoulders and arms for example push-in movement (Kerr & Ness, 2006). This movement stated with the body counter-rotated right side of the body is behind the left side (with respect to the direction of ball trajectory). Similar findings was described by Mc Laughlin (1997). Kerr found that pelvic and shoulder girdle maximum angular velocities occurred concurrently from left arm to the right arm. Many published studies focused on many components of field hockey like the hit (Burges-Limerick et al., 1991), the push (Alexander, 1983), the slap shot (Cresswell & Elliott, 1987), the push-in and trap phases of the penalty corner (Kerr & Ness, 2006), describing specificity of characteristic movements, which could appeared in athletes morphology.

Krzykała (2010) studied the effects of specific one-side dominant training on morphological asymmetry, on the basic of twenty competitive male field hockey players 18-34 years of age. All athletes had played representative hockey at a senior (national) polish level of the game. Average training years of all competitors was 17 y and hesitated between 13 y and 24 y. The anthropometric characteristics in both sides of the body was done by dual energy x-ray absorptiometry, using LUNAR PRODIGY ADVANCE (GE, Madison, WI, USA) densitometer with enCORE software (GE Helthcare v.10.50.086). There were significant differences in body mass density of the legs (1.576 ± 0.0909 g/cm^2 vs. 1.611 ± 0.1062 g/cm^2, respectively: p= 0.0086) and of the trunk (1.111 ± 0.0609 g/cm^2 vs. 1.137 ± 0.0729 g/cm^2, respectively: p=0.0008). In turn there were no differences between right arm 1.017 g/cm^2 and for left arm 1.014 g/cm^2 as well as between total bone mineral density (the right and the left sides of the body) (1.326 ± 0.0741 g/cm^2 vs. 1.338 ± 0.0754 g/cm^2, respectively: p=0.1310). The larger amount of body density was in the left legs, left trunk and total body of athletes. The individual differences between the left and right sides of a particularly body segment show that the biggest diversity among them was in the case of legs. Significant differences in side-to-side lean morphology were observed in every measured parameter. The lean of the arms, legs, trunk and total was higher in the left side of the body. The lean of right arm was 3738 ± 454.9 g vs. 4046 ± 420.7 g for left arm respectively (p=0.0000), lean of right leg was 10578 ± 1050.9 g vs. 10904 ± 1054.5 g, respectively (p=0.0000). Also lean amount was larger in the left side of trunk in comparison to the right (difference: 14371 ± 1580.6 g to 13996 ± 1436.7 g). Significance difference was observed in total lean (30444 ± 2759.5 g for right vs. 31208 ± 2814.5 g for left total, respectively (p=0.0073). There was clear similarity in arms and legs among field hockey players, as opposed to the trunk and total LEAN. Similar findings were observed in a case of body fat analyzing. Across all body segments, the amount of morphological asymmetry was significantly greater in the left side of the body.

In a study of thirty competitive young adult Rugby Union players, Bell et al (2005) observed the arm-lower body contrast in lean soft tissue mass suggesting, that upper and lower limbs contribute equally to playing performance. Also bone mineral mass (BMM) was different according to playing position. The legs were dominant in forwards (-0.76) and the trunk in backs (0.67). The measurements were done using DXA (Hologic QDR/1000W. software version V5.73). Using DXA (QDR-1500, Hologic Corporation, Waltham, MA) in ten healthy postmenopausal tennis players Sanchis-Moysi et al (2004) observed linear relationship between the extent of years of training and the magnitude of the inter-arm difference in bone size- participation in tennis after menarche is connecting with greater bone size and mass in the loaded arm. Some data suggested also that muscle mass is independent predictor of regional and total BMD on the example of gymnasts and elite swimmers with DXA method (Taaffe et al., 1995). Also Calbet et al (2001) study showed a high correlation between the BMD and the muscle mass in the left leg among 33 right-leg dominant male soccer players. Nevil et al (2003) considered the effects of specific training on BMD asymmetry between arms and legs among Caucasians athletes from ten sport disciplines (runners, cyclists, triathletes, racket players, rock climbers, swimmers, rugby players, rowers, kayakers and bodybuilders), at a university or higher level, trained for a minimum of four hour per week, for a minimum of three years. Using DXA on a Hologic QDR 1000W (Bedford, MA) scanner they stated that the differences between the dominant and non-dominant arms were significant but different depends on sport. For example it was greater in the racket players and lesser in the rowers. In the case of right and left legs, there was no asymmetric difference in BMD between them for all athletes combined nor within individual sport disciplines.

The McClanahan et al (2002) study investigated the effects of participation in different sports (NCAA Division I-A baseball, basketball, football, golf, soccer, tennis, cross-country, indoor/outdoor track and volleyball) on side-o-side diversification in bone mineral density (BMD) of the upper and lower limbs. On the basic of 184 collegiate athletes both sexes, and using dual energy X-ray absorptiometry, they revealed greater BMD of the right arms compared with the left arms for all teams. The largest differences were found in the case of men's and women's tennis and men's baseball. The differences in the lower limbs were less common in men and no significant in women.

One limb performance during some certain activities causes its higher fitness level than another limb. Thus training limb become dominate limb, in spite of athletes predisposition to right handedness, left handedness or ambidextratity (Starosta, 1990). Chilibeck et al (2000) asked the question if more bone deposition is a result of greater use of dominant limbs during physical activity or it is connected with fact that the dominant limb is genetically larger. They noticed, using dual energy x-ray absorptiometry, that a greater lifetime of preferential loading of the dominant arm is connected with a greater differences between arms in older group. Also earlier research reported greater mineralization for the dominant humerus but not for dominant radius and ulna, compared to the non-dominant ones, among baseball players 8-19 years of age (Watson, 1973). Additionally, they observed differences in the mineral content between the dominant and non-dominant increasing with age. Tomkinson study show that the increased metabolic rate that accompanies training will tend to increase fluctuating asymmetry in males athletes, at least if the training were conducted during the athlete's growth phase, when disturbances will have the greatest effect (Tomkinson et al., 2003).

3. Conclusion

All above information indicate that DXA is suitable method in athlete study. It allows to gain many valid data about not only overall but also regional body composition. Additionally it is precious method in longitudinal study of body composition assessment, tracking regional changes of some tissues during training program.

That kind of information could be important in a better understanding morphological characteristics of athletes, talent development, sports results improvement and with some injuries prevention. Further longitudinal research in this area could provide deeper insight into characteristic responses on specific training that require asymmetrical limb (side of body) use. Information about side-to-side differences in bone density may be valid for example for strength and conditioning professionals who want to include bilateral training programs minimizing stress-related injuries and maximizing sport results (McClanahan et al., 2002). It could be important to individualized symmetrization process among the athletes, because they do not have the same level of morphological differences. It is obvious that this process should be done methodologically (Starosta, 1990). After the few first stages, movements symmetrization could be used during training and the competitions, what could give quite big advantage over the opponents during the game. It relays on development through the training less fit side of the body and preservation harmony between symmetrical and asymmetrical movement (motor) preparation (Starosta, 1990).

4. References

Abrahao, MRA. & Mello, D. (2008). Anthropometric differences between the right and the left hemi-body of tennis instructor adults and children beginners in the sport and incidence of standard postural deviation. *Fitness Performance Journal*, Vol.7, No.4, pp. 264-270.

Absauomov, TM. et al. (1976). Kontraktionsgeschwin-digkeit von Muskeln und Ihre Veranderung im sportlichen Training. *Leistungssport*, Vol.1, pp. 58-61.

Al-Eisa, E.; Egan, D. & Wassersug, R. (2004). Fluctuating asymmetry and low back pain. *Evolution and Human Behavior*, Vol.25, pp. 31-37.

Alexander, M. (1983). The footwork pattern in the push stroke. *Counterattack*, Vol.3, No. 1, pp. 14-18.

Andreoli, A.; Scalzo, G.; Masala, S.; Tarantino, U. & Guglielmi, G. (2009). Body composition assessment by dual-energy X-ray absprptiometry (DXA). *Radiologia Medica*, Vol.114, pp. 286-300.

Auerbach, BM. & Ruff, CB. (2006). Limb bone bilateral asymmetry: variability and commonality among modern humans. *Journal of Human Evolution*, Vol.50, pp. 203-218.

Bell, W. (2005). The regional placement of bone mineral mass, fat mass, and lean soft tissue mass in young adult Rugby Union players. *Ergonomics*, Vol.48, No.11-14, pp. 1462-1472. ISSN 0014-0139 print / ISSN 1366-5847 online.

Broca, P. (1865). Sur le siege de la Faculte du langage articule. *Bulletin de la Societe de Anthropologie* (Paris), Vol.6, pp. 377- 393.

Bubanj, S. & Obradovic, B. (2002). Mechanical Force and Bones Density, Facta Universitatis. Series:Physical Education and Sport, Vol.1, No.9, pp. 37-50.

Buckley, DC.; Kudsk, KA.; Rose, BA.; Fatzinger, P.; Koetting, CA. & Schlatter, M. (1987). Anthropometric and computed tomography measurements of lower extremity lean body mass. *Journal of the American Dietetic Association*, Vol.87, pp. 196-199.

Burgess-Limerick, R.; Abernethy, B. & Neal, RJ. (1991). Experience and back swing movement time variability: a short note concerning a serendipitous observation. *Human Movement Science*, Vol.10, pp. 621-627.

Buskirk, ER.; Andersen, KL. & Brozek, J. (1956). Unilateral activity and bone and muscle development in the forearm. *Research Quarterly*, Vol.27, pp. 127-131.

Bussey, MD. (2010). Does the demand for asymmetric functional lower body postures in lateral sports related to structural asymmetry of the pelvis. *Journal of Science & Medicine in Sport*, Vol.13, pp. 360-364.

Calbet, JA.; Moysi, JS.; Dorado, C.; Rodriguez, LP. (1998). Bone mineral content and density in professionals tennis players. *Calcified Tissue International*, Vol.62, pp. 491-496.

Calbet, JAL.; Dorado, C.; Diaz-Herrera, P. & Rodriguez-Rodriguez, LP. (2001). High femoral bone mineral content and density in male football (soccer) players. *Medicine and Science in Sports and Exercise*, Vol.33, No.10, pp. 1682-1687.

Chen, Z.; Wang, Z.; Lohman, T. et al. (2007). Dual-energy X-ray absorptiometry is a valid tool for assessing skeletal muscle mass in older women. *Journal of Nutrition*, Vol.137, pp. 2775-2780.

Chettle, DR. & Fremlin, JH. (1984). Techniques of in vivo neutron activation analysis. *Physics in Medicine and Biology*, Vol.29, pp. 1011-1043.

Chhibber, SR. & Singh, I. (1970). Asymmetry in muscle weight and one sided dominance in the human lower limbs. *Journal of Anatomy*, Vol.106, pp. 553-556.

Chilibeck, PD.; Davison, KS.; Sale, DG.; Webber, CE. & Faulkner, RA. (2000). Effect of physical activity on bone mineral density assessed by limb dominance across the lifespan. *American Journal of Human Biology*, Vol.12, No. 5, pp. 633-637.

Chinn, CJ.; Priest, JD. & Kent, BE. (1974). Upper extremity range of motion, grip strength, and girth in highly skilled tennis players. *Physical Therapy*, Vol.54, pp. 474-482.

Cresswell, A. & Elliott, B. (1987). The slap shot or drive in field hockey: a dilemma. *Sport Coach*, Vol.9, pp. 21-23.

Cronin, J. (2010). Leg Asymmetries During Running in Australia Rulet Football Players With Previous Hamstring Injuries. *Journal of Strength & Conditioning Research,* Vol.24, Suplement 1,1.

Czachowska-Sieszycka, B. (1983). Funkcjonalna asymetria mózgu. W: *Biologiczne podstawy zaburzeń psychoruchowego rozwoju dziecka.* Red. Budohoska, W. Warszawa.

De Lorenzo, A.; Bertini, I.; Candeloro, N.; Iacopino, L.; Andreoli, A. & Van Loan, MD. (1998). Comparison of different techniques to measure body composition in moderately active adolescents. *British Journal of Sports Medicine,* Vol.32, pp. 215-219.

Dorado, C.; Sanches Moysi, J.; Vicente, G.; Serrano, JA.; Rodriguez, LP. & Calbet, JAL. (2002). Bone mass, bone mineral density and muscle mass in professional golfers. *Journal of Sports Science,* 20, pp. 591-597.

Ducher, G.; Courteix, D.; Meme, S. et al. (2005). Bone geometry in response to long-term tennis playing and its relationship with muscle volume: a quantitative magnetic resonance imaging study in tennis players. *Bone,* Vol.37, No.4, pp. 457-466.

Egan, DA.; Cole, J. & Twomey, L. (1995). An alternative method for the measurement of pelvic skeletal asymmetry and the association between asymmetry and back pain. In: *M. D'Amico, A. Merolli, G. Santabrogio, Editors, Three dimensional analysis of spinal deformities,* IOS Press, Washington, DC, pp. 171-177.

Ellis, KJ. (2000). Human Body composition: in vivo methods. *Physiological Review,* Vol.80, pp. 649-680.

en.wikipedia.org

Engler, G. (2005). Einstain, his theories, and his aesthetic considerations. *International Studies in the Philosophy Science,* Vol.19, pp. 21-30.

Forbes, GB.; Brown, M. & Griffiths, HJB. (1988). Arm muscle plus bone area: anthropometric and CAT scan compared. *American Journal of Clinical Nutrition,* Vol.47, pp. 929-931.

Faulkner, KG. (2006). Accuracy and precision of the Lunar iDXA, a new fan-beam densitometer. *Journal of Clinical Densitometry,* Vol.9, No.2, pp. 237.

Frey, D. (1949). Zum Problem der Symmetrie in der bildenden Kunst. *Studium Generale,* Vol.2, pp. 268-278.

Fuller, NJ. & Elia, M. (1989). Potential use of bioelectrical impedance of "whole body" and of body segments for the assessment of body composition: A comparison with densitometry and anthropometry. *European Journal of Clinical Nutrition,* Vol.43, pp. 779-791.

Gould, JL. &Gould, CG. (1989). *Sexual selection.* Scientific American Library. New York.

Graham, JH.; Freeman, DC. & Emlen, JM. (1993). Antisymmetry, directional asymmetry, and dynamic morphogenesis. *Genetica,* Vol.89, pp. 121-137.

Grobbelaar, HW. & de Ridder, Hans. (2000). Asymmetry in the upper body of high school fast bowlers in cricket, *2000 Pre-Olympic Congress Sports Medicine and Physical Education. International Congress on Sport Science,* Brisbane, Australia, September 2000.

Haapasalo, H.; Kannus, P.; Sivanen, H.; Pasanen, M.; Uusirasi, K.; Heinonen, A. et al. (1998). Effect of long-term unilateral activity on bone mineral density of female junior tennis players. *Journal of Bone and Mineral Research,* Vol.13, pp. 310-9.

Haarbo, J.; Gotfredsen, A.; Hassager, C. & Christiansen, C. (1991). Validation of body composition by dual energy X-ray absorptiometry (DEXA). *Clin Physiol,* Vol.11, pp. 331-41.

Hargittai, M. & Hargittai, I. (2005). Symmetry in chemistry. *European Review,* Vol.13, No.2, pp. 51-75. Academia Europeans, United Kingdom.

Henche, SA.; Torres, RR. & Pellico, LG. (2008). An evaluation of patterns of change in total and regional body fat mass in healthy Spanish subjects using dual-energy X-ray absorptiometry (DXA). *European Journal of Clinical Nutrition*, Vol.62, pp. 1440-1448.

Hetland, ML.; Haarbo, J. & Christianen, C. (1998). Regional body composition determined by dual-energy x-ray absorptiometry. Relation to training, sex hormones, and serum lipids in male long-distance runners. *Scandinavian Journal of Medicine and Science in Sports*, Vol.8, pp. 102-108.

Heyward, VH. & Wagner, DR. (2004). *Applied body composition assessment*. Sd edition. Human Kinetics.

Jacobsen, T; Schubotz, RI. & Hofer, L. (2006). Brain correlates of aesthetic judgment of beauty. *NeuroImage*, Vol.29, pp. 276-285.

Jones, H.; Priest, J.; Hayes, W.; Tichenor, C. et al. (1977). Humeral hypertrophy in response to exercise. *Journal of Bone and Joint Surgery*, 59a, pp. 204-208.

Jordao, AA.; Bellucci, AD.; Dutra de Oliveira, JE. & Marchini, JS. (2004). Midarm computerized tomography fat, muscle and total areas correlation with nutritional assessment data. *International Journal of Obesity*, Vol.28, pp. 1451-1455.

Kerr, R. & Ness, K. (2006). Kinematics of the Field Hockey Penalty Corner Push-in. *Sports Biomechanics*, Vol.5, No.1, pp. 47-61.

Kimura, K. & Asaeda, S. (1974). On the morphological and functional laterality in human extremities, especially in the lower limb. *Journal of the Anthropological Society of Nippon*, Vol.1982, pp. 189-207.

King, JW.; Grelsford, HJ. & Tullos, HS. (1969). Analysis of the pitching arm of the professional baseball pitcher. *Clinical Orthopedics*, Vol.67, pp. 116-123.

Kistorp, CN.; Toubro, S.; Astrup, A. & Svendsen, OL. (2000). Measurements of body composition by dual-energy x-ray absorptiometry improve prediction of energy expenditure. *Annals of the New York Academy of Science*, Vol.904, No.1, pp. 79-84.

Kohrt, WM. (1995). Body composition by DXA: tried and true? *Medicine and Science in Sports and Exercise*, Vol.27, pp.1349-53.

Komi, PV. (1996).Strength and Power in Sport, in: volume III of The Encyclopedia of Sports Medicine (284-88). Blackwell science.

Koszczyc, T. (1991). *Asymetria morfologiczna I dynamiczna oraz możliwości jej kształtowania u dzieci w młodszym wieku szkolnym*. Studia i Monografie. AWF Wrocław. Poland.

Krawczyk, B.; Skład, M.; Majle, B. & Jackiewicz, A. (1998). Lateran asymmetry in upper and lower limb measurements in selected groups of male athletes. *Biology of Sport*, Vol.15, No.1, pp. 33-38.

Kruger, A.; de Ridder, H.; Underhay, C. & Grobbelaae, H. (2005). Die voorkoms van morfologiese asimmetrie by aliteinternasionale manlike spiesgooiers. *South African Journal for Research in Sport, Physical Education and Recreation*, Vol.27, No.2, pp. 47-55.

Kucera, K. & Henn, S. (2003). Pravention und physiotherapie von verletzungen und uberlastungsschaden im fechten. *Sport Orthopedy and Traumatoly*, Vol.19, pp. 273-280.

Krzykała, M. (2010). Location of body fat by Dual-Energy X-Ray Absorptiometry in professional male field hockey players in relation to their field position. *Studies in Physical Culture and Tourism*, XVI, 2: 179-184.

Lohman, TG. & Chen, Z. (2005). Dual-Energy X-Ray Absorptiometry. In *Human Body Composition* (2nd ed: 63-77). Champaign, IL:Human Kinetics.

Lucki, N. (2006). Physiological Adaptations of the Upper Limb to the Biomechanical Environment of Playing Tennis. *Proceedings of The National Conference On Undergraduate Research.* The University of North Carolina at Asheville.

Lucki, N. & Nicolay, CW. (2007). Phenotypic Plasticity and Fuctional Asymmetry in Response to Grip Forces Exterted by Intercollegiate Tennis Players. *American Journal of Human Biology,* Vol.19, pp. 566-577.

Lukaski, HC. (1987). Methods for the assessment of human body composition: traditional and new. *American Journal of Clinical Nutrition,* Vol.46, pp. 537-56.

Malina, RM. (1979). The effects of exercise on specific tissues, dimensions, and functions during growth. *Studies in Physical Anthropology,* Vol.5, pp. 21-52.

Malina, RM. (1983). Human growth, maturation, and regular physical activity. *Acta Medica Auxologica,* Vol.15, pp. 5-27.

Malina, RM.; Bouchard, C. & Bar-Or, O. (2004). Growth, Maturation and Physical Activity. Human Kinetics.

Malinowski A. (2004). *Auksologia. Rozwój osobniczy człowieka w ujęciu biomedycznym.* Zielona Góra. Poland.

Manning, JT. (1995). Fluctuating asymmetry and body weight in men and women: implications for sexual selection. *Ethology and Sociobiology,* Vol.16, pp. 145-153.

Manning, JT. & Pickup LJ. (1998). Symmetry and performance in middle distance runners. *International Journal of Sports Medicine,* Vol.19, pp. 205-209.

Manning , JT,: Gage, AR.; Diver, MJ.; Scutt, D. & Fraser, WD. (2002). Short-Term Changes in Asymmetry and Hormones in Men. *Evolution and Human Behaviour,* Vol. 23, pp. 95-42.

Marchwicki, I. (1927). Obwody ramienia I przedramienia oraz ich asymetria u chłopców polskich w wieku od 9 do 19 lat. *Przegląd Antropologiczny,* tom II. Poland.

Mascie-Taylor, CGN.; MacLarnon, AM.; Lanigan, PM. & McManus, IC. (1981). Foot-length asymmetry, sex, and handedness. *Science,* Vol.212, pp. 1416-1417.

Maughan, RJ.; Abel, RW.; Watson, JS. & Weir, J. (1986). Forearm Composition and Muscle Function in Trained and Untrained Limbs. *Clinical Physiology,* Vol.6, pp. 389- 396.

McClanahan, BS.; Harmon -Clayton, K.; Ward, KD.; Klesges, RC.; Vukadinovich, CM. & Cantler, ED. (2002). Side-to-side comparisons of bone mineral density in upper and lower limbs of collegiate athletes. *Journal of Strength and Conditioning Research,* Vol.16, No.4, pp. 586-590.

McGrew, WC. & Marchant, LF. (1997). On the other hand: current issue in and meta-analysis the behavioral laterality of hand function in nonhuman primates. *Yearbook of Physical Anthropology,* Vol.40, pp. 201-232.

McLaughlin, P. (1997). Three-dimensional biomechanical analysis of the hockey drag flick. Full report to the Australian Sports Commission. Belconnen: Australian Sports Commision.

Moreno, LA.; Rodriquez, G.; Guillen, J.; Rabanaque, MJ.; Leon, JF. & Arino, A. (2002). Anthropometric measurements in both sides of the body in the assessment of nutritional status in prepubertal children. *European Journal of Clinical Nutrition,* Vol.56, pp. 1208-1215.

Muller, A. (2003). Chemistry: The beauty of symmetry. *Science,* 300, pp. 749-750.

Munter, AH. (1936). A study of the lengths of the long bones of the arms and legs in man, with special reference to Anglo-Saxon skeletons. *Biometrika,* Vol.28, pp. 258-294.

Nevill, MA.; Holder, RL. & Steward, AD. (2003). Modeling elite male athlete's peripheral bone mass, assessed using regional dual x-ray absorptiometry. *Bone,* Vol.32, pp. 62-68.

Nystrom, J.; Lindwall, O.; Ceci, R.; Harmenberg, J.; Svadenhag, J. & Ekblom, B. (1990). Physiological and morphological characteristics of world class fencers. *International Journal of Sports Medicine*, Vol.11, No. 2, pp. 136-139.

O'Connor, MK. (2006). Evaluation of the new Lunar iDXA bone densitometer. *Journal of Clinical Densitometry*, Vol.9, No.2, pp. 237.

Organ, LW.; Bradham, GB.; Gore, DT. & Lozier, SL. (1994). Segmental bioelectrical impedance analysis: Theory and application of a new technique. *Journal of Applied Physiology*, Vol.77, pp. 98-112.

Palmer, AR. & Strobeck, C. (1992). Fluctuating asymmetry as a measure of developmental stability: implications of non-normal distributions and power of statistical tests. *Acta Zoologica Fennica*, Vol.191, pp. 57-72.

Petersen, HL.; Peterson, CT.; Reddy, MB.; Hanson, KB.; Swain, JH.; Sharp, RL. & Alekel, DL. (2006). Body composition, dietary intake, and iron status of female collegiate swimmers and divers. *International Journal of Sport Nutrition and Exercise Metabolism*, Vol.16, pp. 281-295.

Pietrobelli, A.; Wang, Z.; Formica, C. et al. (1998). Dual-energy X-ray absorptiometry: fat estimation errors due to variation in soft tissue hydration. *American Journal of Physiology*, 1988, 274: 808-816.

Pietrobelli, A.; Formica, C.; Wang, Z. & Heymsfield, SB. (1996). Dual-energy X-ray absorptiometry body composition model: Review of physical concepts. *American Journal of Physiology*, Vol.271, pp. E941-E951.

Prives, MG. (1969). Influence of labor and sport upon skeletal structure in man. *Anatomical Record*, Vol.136, No.261.

Roi, GS. & Bianchedi, D. (2008). The Science of Fencing. Implications for Performance and Injury Prevention. *Sports Medicine*, Vol.38, No.6, pp. 465-481.

Ruff, CB.; Walker, A. & Trinkaus, E. (1994). Postcranial robusticity in Homo. III Ontogeny. *American Journal of Physical Anthropology*, 93, pp. 35-54.

Sanchis-Moysi, J.; Dorado, C.; Vicente-Rodriguez, G.; Milutinovic, L.; Garces, GL. & Calbet, JAL. (2004). Inter-arm asymmetry in bone mineral content and bone area in postmenopausal recreational tennis players. *Maturitas*, Vol.48, pp. 289-298.

Schell, LM.; Johnson, FE.; Smith, DR. & Paolone, AM. (1985). Directional asymmetry of body dimension among white adolescents? *American Journal of Physical Anthropology*, Vol.67, pp. 317-322.

Scheltinge, MR.; Jacobs, D.; Kimbrough, TD. & Wilmore, DW. (1991).Alternations in Body Fluid Content Can Be Detected by Bioelectrical Impedance Analysis. *Journal of Surgical Research*, Vol.50, pp. 461-468.

Singh, I. (1970). Functional asymmetry in the lower limbs. *Acta Anatomica*, Vol.77, pp. 131- 138.

Speiser, PW.; Rudolf, MCJ.; Anhalt, H.; Camacho-Hubner, C.; Chiarelli, F.; Eliakim, A. et al. (2005). Consensus statement:n childhood obesity. *Journal of Clinical Endocrinology and Metabolism*, Vol.90, pp. 1871-1887.

Starosta, W. (1990). *Symmetry and asymmetry of movements in sport*. Institutute of Sport, Warsaw, Poland.

Steward, AD. & Hannan, WJ. (2000a). Sub-Regional Tissue Morphometry in Male Athletes and Controls Using Dual X- Ray Absorptiometry (DXA). *International Journal of Sport Nutrition and Exercise Metabolism*, Vol.10, pp. 157-169.

Steward, AD. & Hannan WJ. (200b). Prediction of fat and fat-free mass in male athletes using X-ray absorptiometry as the reference method. *Journal of Sports Sciences*, Vol.18, No.1, pp. 263-274.

The New Lexicon Webster's Encyclopedic Dictionary of the English Language. Deluxe Edition. 1991. Lexicon Publications, Inc. New York.

Taafe, DR.; Snow-Harter, C.; Connolly, DA.; Robinson, TL.; Brown, MD. & Marcus, R. (1995). Differential effects of swimming versus weight-bearing activity on bone mineral status of amenorrhea athletes. *Journal of Bone and Mineral Research*, Vol.10, No.4, pp. 586-593.

Tarociński, A. (1977). Kształtowanie się asymetrii morfologicznej i funkcjonalnej u młodzieży uprawiającej tenis ziemny. *Wychowanie Fizyczne i Sport*, Vol.2, pp. 41-46.

Tomkinson, GR.; Popovic, N. & Martin, M. (2003). Bilateral symmetry and the competitive standard attained in elite and sub-elite sport. *Journal of Sports Science*, Vol.21, pp. 201-211.

Tothill, P.; Arenell, A. & Reid, DM. (1994). Precision and accuracy of measurements of whole-body bone mineral: comparison between Hologic, Lunar and Norland dual energy X-ray absorptiometers. *British Journal of Radiology*, Vol.67, pp. 1210- 1217.

Tsolakis, CH.; Bogdanis, GC. & Vagenas, G. (2006). Anthropometric profile and limb asymmetries in young male and female fencers. *Journal of Human Movement Studies*, Vol. 5, pp. 201-216.

Ulijaszek, SJ. & Mascie-Taylor, CGN. (2005). Anthropometry: the individual and the population, Chapter 2, 2nd, New York. Cambridge University Press.

Watson, RC. (1973). Bone growth and physical activity in young males, Unpublished doctoral dissertation, Madison: University of Wisconsin.

Webber, CE. (1995). Dual photon transitions measurements of bone mass and body composition during growth. In: C Blimke, Jr, O Bar-Or (eds), *New Horizons in Pediatric Exercise Science*. Champaign, IL: Human Kinetics: 57-76.

Wilk, KJ.; Meister, K. & Andrews, JR. (2002). Current concepts in the rehabilitation of the overhead throwing athlete. *American Journal of Sports Medicine*, Vol.31, No.1, pp. 136-51.

Wilmore, JH.; Frisancho, RA.; Gordon, CC.; Himes, JH.; Martin, AD.; Martorell, R. & Seefeldt, RD. (1988). Body breadth equipment and measurement techniques. In *Anthropometric standardization reference manual*, ed. TG. Lohman, AF Roche, and R. Martorell, pp. 27- 38. Champaign: Human Kinetics.

Wolański, N. (1955). Z badań nad tak zwaną maksymalną siłą mięśniową dłoni człowieka i wartość tego pomiaru dla praktyki wychowania fizycznego. *Kultura Fizyczna*, Vol.2. Poland.

Wolański, N. (1962). Wpływ funkcji kończyn (boczności) na kształtowanie asymetrycznej budowy ciała w aspekcie onto- i filogenezy. *Przegląd Antropologiczny*, XXVIII, 1, pp. 27-59. Poland.

www.rjlsystem.com/pdf-files/segmental_bia.pdf

Van Dillen, LR.; Bloom, NJ.; Gombatto, SP. & Susco, TM. (2008). Hip rotation range of motion in people with and without low back pain who participate in rotation-related sports. *Physical Therapy in Sport*, Vol. 9, pp. 72-81.

Van Dusen, CR. (1939). An anthropometric study of the upper extremities of children. *Human Biology*, Vol.11, pp. 277-284.

Van Valen, A. (1962). A study of fluctuating asymmetry. *Evolution*, Vol. 16, pp. 125-142.

Zeidel, DW. & Hessamian, M. (2010). Asymmetry and Symmetry in the Beauty of Human Faces. *Symmetry*, Vol.2, pp. 136-149.

6

Body Composition in Disabilities of Central Nervous System

Yannis Dionyssiotis[1,2]
[1]*Physical and Social Rehabilitation Center Amyntæo*
[2]*University of Athens, Laboratory for Research of the Musculoskeletal System*
Greece

1. Introduction

Disability leads to immobilisation associated with profound changes in body composition. The potential risks involved with these changes i.e. loss of lean tissue mass (LM) and bone mineral density (BMD) vs. gain in fat mass (FM) in body composition have implications for the health of the disabled individuals (Jones et al., 1998). Body fat has been identified as a significant predictor of mortality in humans making body composition measurement to quantify nutritional and health status an important issue for human health. (Seidell et al., 1996; Bender et al., 1998; Van Der Ploeg et al., 2003). Moreover, some disorders such as carbohydrate intolerance, insulin resistance, lipid abnormalities, and heart disease occur prematurely and at a higher prevalence in disabled populations may be related to adverse changes in body composition that result from immobilization and skeletal muscle denervation (Spungen et al., 2003).

In traumatic and pathological lesions of the central nervous system (CNS) there are differences according to the evolution or not of the lesion (i.e. progressive multiple sclerosis vs. complete paraplegia), the type of injury (i.e. lesion with a level of injury vs. upper motor neuron pyramidal lesion), life expectancy, the residual mobility and functionality, the ability to walk and stand (i.e. incomplete paraplegia vs. quadriplegia vs. high-low paraplegia) and drug treatment (i.e. frequent corticosteroid therapy in multiple sclerosis vs. long-term therapy with anticoagulants in paraplegia). In addition there are differences in the degree of spasticity which is likely to play a regulatory role in maintaining bone density (Dionyssiotis et al., 2011a). We need to take into account the element of fatigue and muscle weakness in disabilities, especially in diseases like multiple sclerosis, which significantly reduces the mobility of these patients (Krupp et al., 2010).

The relative difference in energy expenditure between individuals with multiple sclerosis (MS) and able-bodied subjects is probably lower than the relative difference in physical activity, because individuals with MS have a higher energy expenditure of physical activity (Olgiati et al., 1988). Reduced physical activity (and probably reduced energy expenditure) in MS need to be accompanied by a reduction in energy intake otherwise body fat will increase (Lambert et al., 2002). Subjects with those motor disorders often face problems of depression and limit mobility (Dionyssiotis, 2011b). Moreover, in children with cerebral palsy (CP) studies suggest that increased stretch reflexes and muscle tone, weakness of involved musculature, and severe limitation of movement reduce the capacity to perform normal movements creating ambulation barriers limiting physical activity. The dependency on mobility devices, common in all disabilities, and the frequent periods of immobilization after multiple operative procedures contribute to the hypoactivity status of such children. It could be assumed that, under these conditions, body composition may be significantly compromised (Chad et al., 2000).

Studies found that lean mass of the contralateral limb was lower compared to the ipsilateral limb in upper motor neuron injury, as occurs in stroke (Ryan et al., 2000; 2002). Similar findings of reduced muscle mass and increased intramuscular fat have been also published in individuals with incomplete spinal cord injury (SCI) (Gorgey et al., 2007) suggesting that reduced muscle mass is fundamentally related to poor fitness and physical performance capacity after stroke (Hafer-Macko et al., 2008).

On the other side the clinical equivalence of diseases with different physiopathology, location, evolution, etc. could be similar; i.e. a severe form of MS can result in a wheelchair bound patient a clinical figure equivalent to paraplegia or a MS patient may have a more appropriate walking gait pattern vs. a patient with incomplete paraplegia but may also be unable to walk at all, is bedridden and vice versa (Dionyssiotis, 2011b; 2011c; 2011d). In addition to these differences and according to osteoporosis the role of factors which do not change, such as race or gender of patients has not been yet clarified, although there are few studies in women debating that bone mass in women with disabilities is more affected than men (Smeltzer et al., 2005; Coupaud et al., 2009).

Therefore, the purpose of this chapter was to present the bone-mineral density, bone-mineral content, and bone-mineral-free lean and fat tissue mass alterations of ambulatory and non-ambulatory subjects with disabilities of the central nervous system.

2. Body composition measurements

2.1 Anthropometric and various techniques of body composition measurements

In a study which investigated a chronic spinal cord injury (SCI) population with paraplegia (Dionyssiotis, 2008a, Dionyssiotis et al., 2008b) values of body mass index (BMI, kg/m^2) did not present statistical significance in relation to the controls, which is a finding in line with the literature (Maggioni et al., 2003; Mamoun et al., 2004).. Nevertheless, there are studies which demonstrate the usefulness of BMI as an indicator of obesity, in body composition in people with spinal cord injury (Gupta et al., 2006). These studies, however, included both tetraplegics and middle-aged people unlike the Greek one which included relatively young individuals (Dionyssiotis et al., 2008a). Whether the criteria of BMI may assess obesity in people with spinal cord injury the latest studies show the opposite (McDonald et al., 2007).

BMI of a male paraplegic group was slightly greater compared to a tetraplegic one and distribution of BMI by level of injury was similar with 37.5% and 40.5% of the male tetraplegic and male paraplegic groups, respectively, falling into the recommended BMI range. Approximately 50% in each male group were overweight by BMI, and 12.5% and 10.8%, respectively, were classified as obese. Overall, when compared with the general population-observed distribution by BMI, a greater proportion of men with SCI fell into the desirable BMI range and fewer fell into the obese category (Groah et al., 2009).

No differences were found in BMI between paraplegics in the acute phase of injury and controls, which is a finding in accordance with other studies in which, despite the same BMI, the body composition and the distribution of fat and fat free mass were altered in patients with spinal cord injury, with the fat free mass being statistically significantly lower in paraplegic patients in total body composition and in the lower, but not the upper limbs. As far as the fat mass is concerned, it was statistically significantly higher (kilograms and %) in the total body composition in the upper and lower limbs (Maimoun et al., 2006).

These findings show that using the BMI does not contribute substantially in determining the body composition of paraplegics and lowers the percentage of fat in this population, finding that agrees with other studies and shows that the anthropometric measurement with BMI in paraplegics, underestimates fat in body composition when measurements are compared with healthy subjects (Jones et al., 1998).

Body mass index is a very simple measurement of fat; however it does not distinguish the individual components of weight. The applicability of conventional BMI cut off values is into question (Buchholz, 2005; McDonald et al., 2007). BMI is an insensitive marker of obesity in subjects with SCI and measuring fat with BMI in chronic paraplegic patients is not enough to determine subject's percentage of fat in the body (Olle et al., 1993).

To standardize or index physiological variables, such as resting metabolic rate and power fat free mass (FFM) is usually used (Van Der Ploeg et al., 2003). Skeletal muscle represents 50% of the non fat component in the total body (Clarys et al., 1984; Modlesky et al., 2004) and exact quantification of the amount of skeletal muscle is important to assess nutritional status, disease risk, danger of illnesses, physical function, atrophic effects of aging, and muscle-wasting diseases (Forbes, 1987; Mojtahedi et al., 2008).

Because muscle wasting is a common sign of cerebral palsy (CP), even in well nourished children, the validity of using muscle wasting as evidence or measurement of malnutrition in CP is in doubt. Studies found that the triceps, midthigh, and calf skinfold thicknesses of the affected side were greater than those of the no affected side among children with hemiplegic CP (Stevenson et al., 1995). Useful information regarding fat provide triceps, subscapular skinfolds and arm-fat area (Patrick & Gisel, 1990). Other studies support the concept that the validity of skinfold thickness as an assessment of limb fat storage is dependent on the preservation of limb muscles (Ingemann-Hansen T et al., 1977) and suggested good sensitivity and specificity of triceps skinfold thickness for predicting mid-upper arm fat area probably were attributable to good preservation of mid-upper arm muscles among children with CP (Samson-Fang et al., 2000).

In disabled children techniques for measuring skinfolds are well established and standardised (Lohman et al., 1988) and equations are available for calculation of body fat from skin fold thickness (Slaughter et al., 1988) although unvalidated in this population, as are normative values for skinfold thickness (Frisancho, 1981; Kuperminc & Stevenson, 2008). Consequently, use of skinfold thickness as a measurement, especially for the affected limb, should be used with discretion in the assessment of children with CP, who tend to have muscle wasting.

In cerebral palsy neither bioelectrical impedance analysis nor predictive equations for skinfold thickness generated from normal, able-bodied adults accurately determined percentage body fat (Hildreth et al., 1997). Body mass index (BMI), triceps skinfold thickness, subscapular skinfold thickness, suprailiac skinfold thickness, and circumferences of the biceps, waist, forearm, and knee were all significantly correlated with percentage body fat (Bandini et al., 1991).

BMI in patients with MS was statistically less compared to age comparable controls (Formica et al., 1997). In a recent study both total body fat and mass percent showed consistent significant dependence from BMI, as among normal subjects. Multiple linear regression analysis of bone mineral percent at all studied sites showed consistent dependence from BMI (increased with higher BMI) for both patient and control groups (Sioka et al., 2011).

Changes in body composition in spinal cord injured subjects can be assessed with various techniques including isotope-labelled water (Jones et al., 1998) total body potassium counting (Lussier et al., 1983; Spungen et al., 1992) anthropometric measures (Bulbulian et al., 1987) hydrodensitometry (Lussier et al., 1983; Sedlock, 1990) dual photon absorptiometry (DPA) (Spungen et al., 1992; Changlai, 1996) and dual energy X-ray absorptiometry (DXA) (Jones et al., 1998). However, some of these methods are not particularly suitable for use in the SCI population.

The hydrodensitometric model was regarded as the "gold standard" for body composition assessment. This model partitions the body into two compartments of constant densities [fat mass: 0.9007 g/cm^3 and FFM: 1.100 g/cm^3] and assumes that the relative amounts of the FFM components [water, protein, protein, bone mineral (BM), and non-BM] are fixed (Brozek et al., 1963; Van Der Ploeg et al., 2003). Hydrodensitometry is clearly inappropriate for individuals who deviate from these fixed and/or assumed values (e.g., children, elderly, blacks, obese), and its application is, therefore, somewhat limited (Womersley et al., 1976; Schutte, 1984; Lohman, 1986; Fuller et al., 1996).

Bioelectrical impedance analysis (BIA) has been used to measure cerebral palsy subjects. However, the inclusion of weight in the BIA predictive equation may reduce its accuracy in determining change in lean body mass (Forbes et al., 1992). The inability of BIA to accurately predict percentage body fat in the sample may be related to several factors. In the BIA method where the impedance of a geometrical system (i.e., the human body) is dependent on the length of the conductor (height) and its configuration, it is almost impossible to measure accurately height in subjects with CP because of their muscle contractures. An over- or underestimation of height by 2.5 cm can result in a 1.0-L error in the estimation of TBW, producing a small error in the estimation of percentage body fat (< 5%). The second major problem is body asymmetry which renders the assumption of a symmetrical configuration of the human body invalid in this case. (National Institutes of Health Technology Assessment Conference Statement, 1994; Hildreth et al., 1997).

Isotope dilution measures the water compartment of the whole body rather than a single area assumed to mimic the composition of the whole body. Thus, the use of a stable isotope to measure body composition is ideal for people with CP because it is non-invasive, does not require the subject to remain still for the measurement, and is independent of height and body symmetry. However, the prohibitive cost of the isotopes and the need for a mass spectrometry facility and highly trained technicians make this method impractical for routine clinical use (Hildreth et al., 1997).

To determine whether bioelectrical impedance analysis and anthropometry can be used to determine body composition for clinical and research purposes in children with cerebral palsy 8 individuals (two female, mean age=10 years, mean gross motor function classification=4.6 [severe motor impairment]) recruited from an outpatient tertiary care setting underwent measurement of fat mass, fat-free mass, and percentage body fat using BIA, anthropometry (two and four skinfold equations), and dual-energy x-ray absorptiometry. Correlation were excellent for determination of fat-free mass for all methods (i.e., all were above 0.9) and moderate for determination of fat mass and percent body fat (range=0.4 to 0.8). Moreover, skinfolds were better predictors of percent body fat, while bioelectrical impedance was a better predictor for fat mass (Liu et al., 2005). On the contrary another study investigated the pattern of body composition in 136 subjects with spastic quadriplegic cerebral palsy, 2 to 12 years of age, by anthropometric measures, or by anthropometric and total body water (TBW) measures (n = 28), compared with 39 control subjects. Body composition and nutritional status indicators were significantly reduced. Calculation of body fat from two skinfolds correlated best with measures of fat mass from TBW (Stallings et al., 1995; Kuperminc & Stevenson, 2008).

Magnetic resonance imaging (MRI) provides remarkably accurate estimates of skeletal muscle in vivo (Modlesky et al., 2004). MRI and also quantitative computed tomography (QCT) have been validated in studies of humancadavers in the assessment of regional skeletal muscle (Mitsiopoulos et al., 1998). Although, these devices have disadvantages of high radiation exposure and are expensive.

2.2 Dual-energy X-ray absorptiometry (DXA)

Recently, dual-energy X-ray absorptiometry (DXA) has gained acceptance as a reference method for body composition analysis (Mahon et al., 2007; LaForgia et al., 2009). Originally designed to determine bone density, DXA technology has subsequently been adopted for the assessment of whole body composition and offers estimation rapidly, non-invasively and with minimal radiation exposure (Van Der Ploeg et al., 2003; Dionyssiotis et al., 2008a). Moreover, is well tolerated in subjects who would be unable to tolerate other body composition techniques, such as underwater weighing (hydro-densitometry) (Laskey, 1996). DXA software determines the bone mineral and soft tissue composition in different regions of the body being a three-compartment model that quantifies: (i) bone mineral density and content (BMD, BMC), (ii) fat mass (FM); and (iii) lean mass (LM), half of which is closely correlated with muscle mass and also yields regional as well as total body values (Rittweger et al., 2000) for example in the arms, legs, and trunk (figure 1).

DXA analyzes differently the dense pixels in body composition. Soft tissue pixels are analyzed for two materials: fat and fat-free tissue mass. Variations in the fat mass/fat free tissue mass composition of the soft tissue produce differences in the respective attenuation coefficients at both energy levels. The ratio at the two main energy peaks is automatically calculated of the X-ray attenuation providing separation of the soft tissue compartment into fat mass and fat-free tissue mass (lean mass) (Peppler & Mazess, 1981; Pietrobelli et al., 1996). A bone-containing pixel is analyzed for "bone mass" (bone mineral content, BMC) and soft tissue as the two materials. Thus, the fat mass/fat free tissue mass of the soft tissue component of the bone pixels cannot be measured, but only estimated (Ferretti et al., 2001).

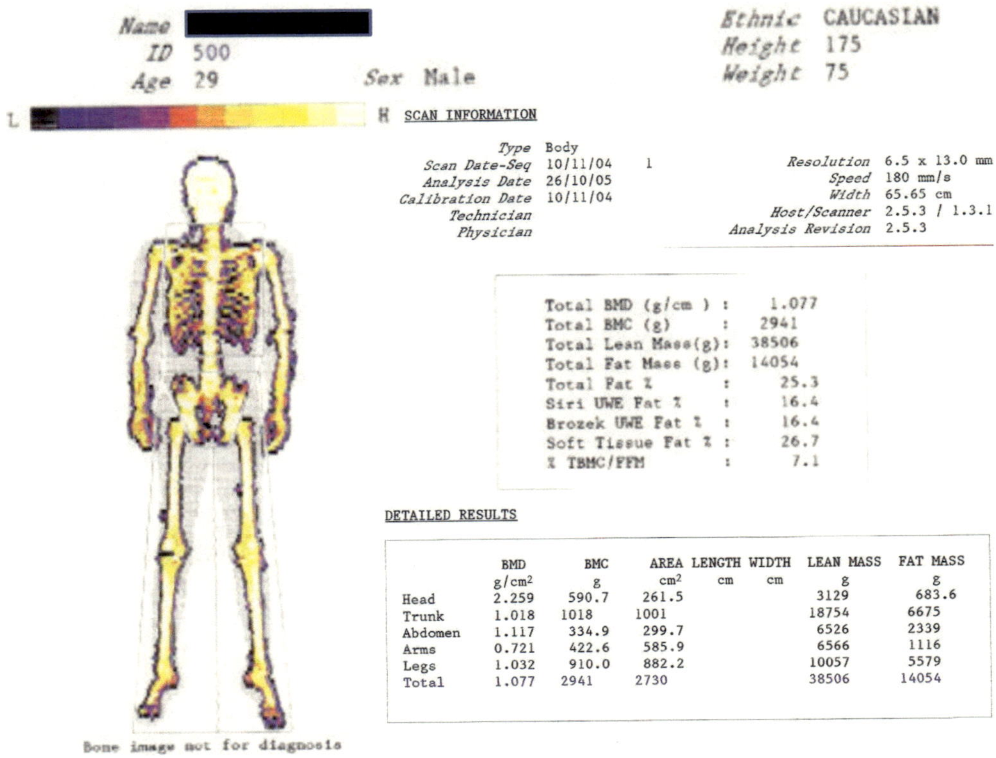

Name [redacted]
ID 500
Age 29 Sex Male

Ethnic CAUCASIAN
Height 175
Weight 75

L H SCAN INFORMATION

Type Body
Scan Date-Seq 10/11/04 1
Analysis Date 26/10/05
Calibration Date 10/11/04
Technician
Physician

Resolution 6.5 x 13.0 mm
Speed 180 mm/s
Width 65.65 cm
Host/Scanner 2.5.3 / 1.3.1
Analysis Revision 2.5.3

Total BMD (g/cm)	:	1.077
Total BMC (g)	:	2941
Total Lean Mass(g)	:	38506
Total Fat Mass (g)	:	14054
Total Fat %	:	25.3
Siri UWE Fat %	:	16.4
Brozek UWE Fat %	:	16.4
Soft Tissue Fat %	:	26.7
% TBMC/FFM	:	7.1

DETAILED RESULTS

	BMD	BMC	AREA	LENGTH	WIDTH	LEAN MASS	FAT MASS
	g/cm²	g	cm²	cm	cm	g	g
Head	2.259	590.7	261.5			3129	683.6
Trunk	1.018	1018	1001			18754	6675
Abdomen	1.117	334.9	299.7			6526	2339
Arms	0.721	422.6	585.9			6566	1116
Legs	1.032	910.0	882.2			10057	5579
Total	1.077	2941	2730			38506	14054

Bone image not for diagnosis

Fig. 1. Whole body and regional distribution of fat mass, lean mass, bone mineral content (BMC) and bone mineral density (BMD) from paraplegic subject thoracic 6 using whole body DXA (Norland X-36, Fort Atkinson, Wisconsin, USA) and values of measured parameters. Modified and translated with permission from Dionyssiotis, 2008a.

The important issue on this is the investigation of distribution of bone mineral, fat and mass throughout the body. These changes induce the risk for diseases such as diabetes, coronary heart disease, dyslipidaimias and osteoporosis (Bauman et al., 1992; Bauman & Spungen, 1994; Kocina, 1997; Garland et al., 1992). There is a need to quantify the alterations in body composition to prevent these diseases and their complications. Studies also reported that bone density measurements at one site cannot usefully predict the bone density elsewhere (Heymsfield et al., 1989) because different skeletal regions, even with similar quantities of trabecular or cortical bone, may respond variably in different physiopathological conditions (Laskey, 1996).

In disabled conditions the accuracy of skeletal muscle measured by DXA may be compromised when muscle atrophy is present. A lower ratio of muscle to adipose-tissue-free mass indicates a lower proportion of muscle in the fat-free soft tissue mass. Cross-sectional area of skeletal muscle in the thighs after SCI is extensively reduced (Castro et al., 1999). If this is the case muscle mass would be overestimated by prediction models that assume that muscle represents all or a certain proportion of the fat-free soft tissue mass, i.e.

in spinal cord injured subjects (Modlesky et al., 2004). DXA technique has been used in assessment of SCI and appears to be tolerated well by this population (Szollar et al., 1997; Uebelhart et al., 1995; Chow et al., 1996).

Name	[redacted]	*Ethnic*	cauc
ID	2210	*Height*	180
Age	36 *Sex* Male	*Weight*	125

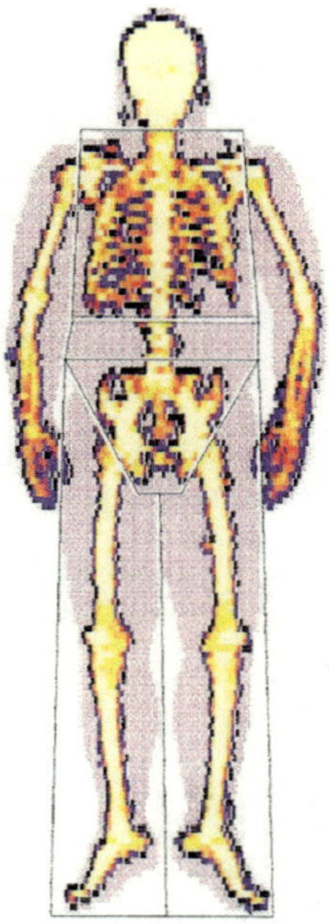

Total BMD (g/cm)	:	1.256
Total BMC (g)	:	3527
Total Lean Mass(g)	:	79838
Total Fat Mass (g)	:	40884
Total Fat %	:	32.9
Siri UWE Fat %	:	29.6
Brozek UWE Fat %	:	28.6
Soft Tissue Fat %	:	33.9
% TBMC/FFM	:	4.2

DETAILED RESULTS

	BMD g/cm2	BMC g	AREA cm2	LENGTH cm	WIDTH cm	LEAN MASS g	FAT MASS g
Head	2.218	586.9	264.6			4142	1035
Trunk	1.254	1181	942.0			40251	24108
Abdomen	1.542	564.3	365.8			17188	12251
Arms	0.781	456.0	583.7			8784	4205
Legs	1.280	1302	1017			26661	11536
Total	1.256	3527	2807			79838	40884

Fig. 2. Whole body and regional distribution of fat mass, lean mass, bone mineral content (BMC) and bone mineral density (BMD) from control male subject using whole body DEXA Norland X-36 and values of measured parameters. Modified and translated with permission from Dionyssiotis, 2008a.

3. Physiopathological context

3.1 Spinal cord injury

Spinal cord injury (SCI) always results in substantial and rapid bone loss predominately in areas below the neurological level of injury. The predominant finding of SCI on bone is a large loss of bone during the first year of injury (Spungen et al., 2003) and an ongoing demineralisation 3 years after trauma in tibia (Biering-Sörensen et al., 1988) with a progressive bone loss over 12 to 16 months prior to stabilizing (Lazo et al., 2001) was demonstrated.

Cancellous bone is more affected than cortical bone after SCI. In a prospective study, six acute tetraplegics were followed up for 12 months, and the trabecular and cortical BMD's of the tibia were found to be decreased by 15 and 7% (Frey-Rindova et al., 2000), while in paraplegics trabecular metaphysical-epiphyseal areas of the distal femur and the proximal tibia are the most affected sites (Jiang et al., 2006). A cross-sectional study (Dauty et al., 2000) in SCI subjects demonstrated a significant demineralization at the distal femur (-52%) and the proximal tibia (-70%), respectively.

There is no demineralization of the upper limbs in paraplegics. Studies reported a minor increase of BMD while at the lumbar spine trabecular bone demineralization remains relatively low compared to long bones cortical bone demineralization of (Dauty et al., 2000). Normal (Chantraine et al., 1986; Biering-Sorensen et al., 1988; Kunkel et al., 1993) or even higher than normal values were found (Ogilvie et al., 1993), a phenomenon known as "dissociated hip and spine demineralization" (Leslie, 1993) One reason for preservation of bone mass in the vertebral column is because of its continued weight-bearing function in paraplegics but also lumbar spine arthrosis, bone callus, vertebral fracture, aortic calcification, osteosynthesis material, etc. Degenerative changes in the spine may be the most possible reason to give falsely higher values of BMD (Dauty et al., 2000).

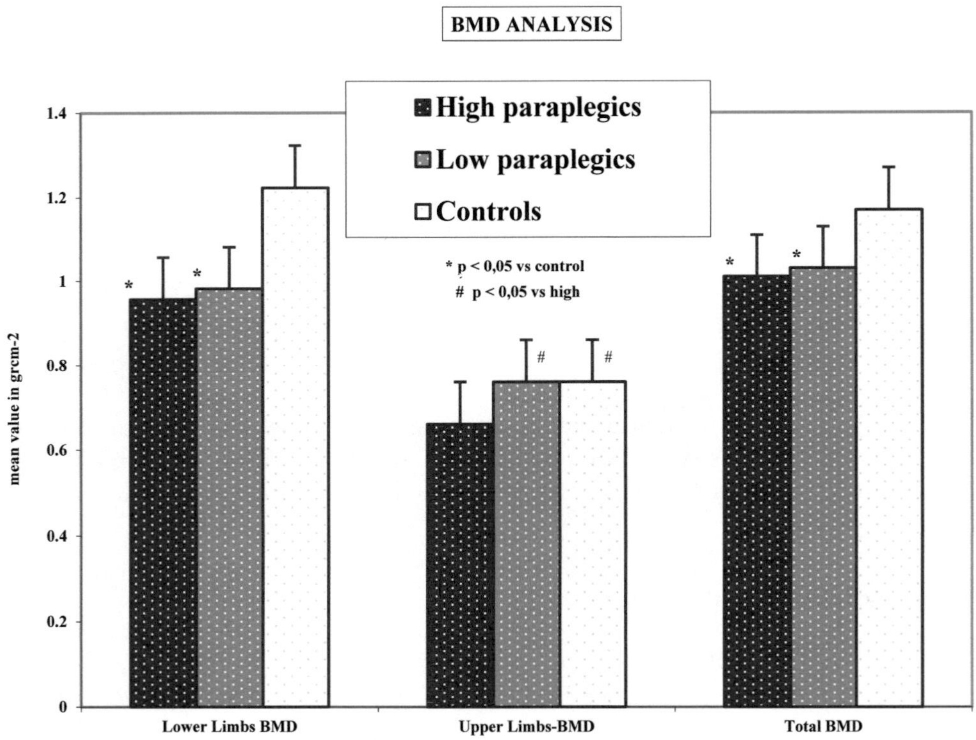

Fig. 3. The picture depicts the analysis of bone mineral density (BMD) in high and low level paraplegics and controls. A statistically significant reduction in total BMD ($p<0.001$) and lower limbs BMD in body composition compared to able-bodied males was observed. On the contrary, upper limbs BMD was higher in low paraplegics and controls, an unexpected finding explained in the paper of Dionyssiotis et al., 2008b. Diagram modified and translated from Dionyssiotis, 2008a.

The neurological level of the lesion i.e. the extent of impairment of motor and sensory function is important, because tetraplegics are more likely to lose more bone mass throughout the skeleton than paraplegics (Tsuzuku et al., 1999). In paraplegics legs' BMC was reduced vs. controls, independently of the neurological level of injury and negatively correlated with the duration of paralysis in total paraplegic group, but after investigation according to the neurological level of injury this correlation was due to the strong correlation of high paraplegics' legs BMC with the duration of paralysis, meaning that the neurological level of injury determines the extent of bone loss (Dionyssiotis et al., 2009). The similar severity of demineralization in the sublesional area was shown between paraplegics and tetraplegics, and the extent of the bone loss may be variable (Demirel et al., 1998; Tsuzuku et al., 1999; Dauty et al., 2000).

The duration of paralysis has an inverse relationship with leg percentage-matched BMD and trunk percentage-matched BMD (Clasey et al., 2004). In addition in complete paraplegics, with high (thoracic 4-7) and low (thoracic 8-12) neurological level of injury, upper limbs FM and lower limbs BMD were correlated with the duration of paralysis in total paraplegic group but after investigation according the neurological level of injury this correlation was due to the strong correlation of high paraplegics' lower limbs BMD with the duration of paralysis. The explanation of this strong correlation could possibly lie on higher incidence of standing in the group of low paraplegics and direct effect of loading lower limbs while standing and walking with orthotic equipment. Moreover, the association of the duration of paralysis with parameters below and above the neurological level of injury (upper limbs FM) raises the question of the existence of a hormonal mechanism as an influential regulator in paraplegics' body composition (Dionyssiotis, 2008a; Dionyssiotis et al., 2008b; 2009).

Actually, little is known regarding the nature and time frame of the influence of complete SCI on human skeletal muscle because published data are coming from cross-sectional studies, where different groups with few subjects have been examined at different times, usually in the chronic phase of paralysis. Disuse was thought to be the mechanism responsible for the skeletal muscle atrophy in paraplegics, but muscle fibres following SCI begin to change their functional properties early post injury. Muscle fiber cross-sectional area (CSA) has been suggested to decline from 1 to 17 months after injury and thereafter to reach its nadir. Conversion to type II fibers has been suggested to occur between 4 months and 2 years after injury, resulting in even slow-twitch muscle becoming predominantly fast twitch thereafter (Castro et al., 1999). Metabolic enzymes levels in skeletal muscle might be expected to be reduced after SCI because of inactivation. In support of this contention, succinic dehydrogenase (SDH) activity, a marker of aerobic-oxidative capacity, has been reported to be 47–68% below control values in fibers of tibialis anterior muscle years after injury in support of this contention (Scelsi, 2001).

The muscle atrophy in SCI is of central type and depends on the disuse and loss of upper connections of the lower motor neuron, sometimes associated to the loss of anterior horn cells and transinaptic degeneration. The last alteration may be responsible for the denervation changes seen in early stages post SCI. In the later stages (10-17 months post SCI) diffuse muscle atrophy with reduction of the muscle fascicle dimension is associated to fat infiltration and endomysial fibrosis. In all stages post SCI, almost all patients showed myopathic changes, as internal nuclei, fibre degeneration and cytoplasmic vacuolation due to lipid accumulation (Scelsi, 2001)

It is evident that other co-factors as spasticity and microvascular damage, contribute to the induction of the marked morphological and enzyme histochemical changes seen in the paralyzed skeletal muscle (Scelsi, 2001). Small fibers, predominantly fast-twitch muscle, and low mitochondrial content have been reported years after injury in cross-sectional studies. These data have been interpreted to suggest that human skeletal muscle shows plasticity (Castro et al., 1999).

On the contrary, force loss during repetitive contractions evoked by surface electrical stimulation (ES) of skeletal muscle in humans does not appear to be altered within a few months of injury (Shields, 1995) but it is greater a year or more after SCI (Hillegass & Dudley, unpublished observations). The greater fatigue, when evident, was partially attributed to lower metabolic enzyme levels (Scelsi, 2001).

Muscular loading of the bones has been thought to play a role in the maintenance of bone density (de Bruin et al., 1999; Dionyssiotis et al., 2011d). However, the ability to stand or ambulate itself does not improve BMD or prevent osteoporosis after SCI.

Controversial results have also been reported regarding the effect of spasticity on BMD in SCI paraplegics. A cross-sectional study of 41 SCI paraplegics reported less reduction of BMD in the spastic paraplegics SCI patients compared to the flaccid paraplegic SCI patients (Demirel et al., 1998). Others reported that spasticity may be protective against bone loss in SCI patients, however, without any preserving effect in the tibia (Dionyssiotis et al., 2011a; Eser et al., 2005). A possible explanation for that could lie in the fact paraplegics to be above thoracic (T)12 level with various degrees of spasticity according to the Ashworth scale. In addition, muscle spasms affecting the lower leg would mainly be extension spasms resulting in plantar flexion thus creating little resistance to the contracting muscles. Furthermore, the measuring sites of the tibia did not include any muscle insertions of either the knee or the ankle extensor muscles (Dionyssiotis et al., 2011a, 2011d). Other investigators also have not been able to establish a correlation between BMD and muscle spasticity (Lofvenmark et al., 2009).

The hormone leptin is secreted by fat cells and helps regulate body weight and energy consumption (Fruhbeck et al., 1998). The percentage of fat in people is positively correlated with the amount of leptin in the circulation (Maffei et al., 1995). In SCI, when compared with healthy subjects, higher levels of leptin have been found, possibly due to greater fat tissue storage (Bauman et al., 1996). Leptin activates the sympathetic nervous system (SNS) through a central administration. The disruption of the sympathetic nervous system i.e. in tetraplegia and high level paraplegia may modify the secretion and activity of the leptin, because the sympathetic preganglionic neurons become atrophic in these subgroups (Elias et al., 1998; Correia et al., 2001) leading to disturbed irritation from leptin below the neurological level of injury. In addition, extensive obesity is known to reduce lipolytic sensitivity (Haque et al., 1999; Horowitz et al., 1999, 2000).

In high level spinal cord injuries there is a disorder of the autonomic nervous system and combined to the fact that the hormone leptin activates the sympathetic nervous system through central control it could be suggested that "the closure of paths" of the central nervous system disrupts the effect of leptin and possibly increases the risk of obesity in SCI subjects with high-level injury (Krassioukov et al., 1999; Jeon et al., 2003). However, after separation of SCI subjects into those with an injury above or below Thoracic (T) 6, leptin levels were significantly higher in the former group. T6 appears to be the lowest level of injury in most patients with SCI to develop autonomic dysreflexia. With SCIs above the level of T6, there is reduced SNS outflow and supraspinal control to the splanchnic outflow and the lower-extremity blood vessels while serum leptin levels in men with SCI correlated not only with BMI but also with the neurologic deficit. This finding supports the notion that decentralization of sympathetic nervous activity relieves its inhibitory tone on leptin secretion, because subjects with tetraplegia have a more severe deficit of sympathetic nervous activity (Wang et al., 2005).

3.2 Multiple sclerosis

No significant difference between ambulatory multiple sclerosis (MS) patients and non MS controls in body composition was found despite lower physical activity in ambulatory MS patients (Lambert et al., 2002). In MS subjects there was no significant relation between any of the body composition measures and the level of disability as measured by the Expanded Disability Status Scale (EDSS). Others found no difference in body fat percent between ambulatory MS patients (Formica et al., 1997) and lower physical activity in ambulatory MS patients vs. controls (Ng & Kent-Braun, 1997). A possible explanation for the similar body composition may be lower energy intake in MS individuals who are ambulatory and greater energy cost of physical activity (walking) in MS than it is with non MS controls (Lambert et al., 2002).

A significant inverse relation between free fat mass (FFM) and EDSS score when ambulatory and non ambulatory MS subjects were combined was found (Formica et al., 1997). On the contrary others without including non ambulatory subjects did not find a significant inverse relation between FFM percent and EDSS score (Lambert et al., 2002). It would seem apparent that ambulatory patients with MS and controls would strengthen the inverse relation between FFM and EDSS score.

The finding of no relation between EDSS score and body fat percent (Lambert et al., 2002) fits well with studies which found no significant relation between the level of physical activity, and the level of disability in individuals with MS (Ng & Kent-Braun, 1997) because MS would likely have a much greater effect on physical activity than on energy intake. According to these findings it appears that the level of disability of ambulatory individuals with MS does not predict body composition. This suggests that a significant level of disability does not force these individuals to be physically inactive and does not result in a greater body fat content. There are many detrimental manifestations of excess body fat, such as hyperlipidemia, insulin resistance, and type II diabetes (Lambert et al., 2002). The largest component of FFM is muscle mass (Lohman, 1986). If muscle mass is lower in individuals with MS than in controls, it may also contribute to the impaired ability to ambulate and perform other activities of daily living. Muscle fiber size from biopsy specimens of the tibialis anterior were 26% smaller than specimens from control subjects (Kent-Braun et al., 1997). Thus, at least for this small muscle, muscle mass was lower in MS. This relationship may not hold for other muscle groups or for whole-body muscle mass (Lambert et al., 2002).

Another reason for skeletal muscle alterations is glucocorticoid usage. The prolonged duration of glucocorticoid causes catabolism of skeletal muscle. Decreased amino acid transport into muscle and increased glutamine synthesis activity with resultant muscle atrophy are some of the concomitant effects of glucocorticoid use on skeletal muscle.

Endogenous glucocorticoid excess also produces generalized osteoporosis, most prevalent in trabecular-rich skeletal regions (Formica et al., 1997).

Beside corticosteroids, immunomodulatory, antiepileptic and antidepressant drugs usually used in individuals with MS, high incidence of vitamin D deficiency, molecular mechanisms and disuse-loss of mechanical stimuli in bone have an effect on bone integrity (most believe that immobilization of these patients is a minor factor in the etiology of osteoporosis) (Dionyssiotis, 2011).

3.3 Stroke

Longitudinal studies of body composition in the elderly have shown that body cell mass decreases with age and is lower in women than in men (Steen et al., 1985). A decline in body fat in both the dependent and independent groups nine weeks after admission was found, indicating consumption of energy stores. In contrast, the change of body cell mass between admission and after 9 weeks was significantly greater in the dependent patients compared with the independent (Unosson et al., 1994). Immobilized individuals lose muscle mass irrespective of nutritional intake because of reduced synthesis of proteins, while the rate of breakdown of proteins is unchanged (Schonheyder et al., 1954). During the recovery period the stroke patients seemed to break down body fat to compensate for energy needs, independent of their functional condition. However, change of body cell mass appeared to relate to the patients' functional condition after stroke (Unosson et al., 1994).

A study in 35 stroke patients compared the body composition, including lean tissue mass, fat tissue mass, and bone mineral content, of the paretic leg with that of the non affected leg in patients with stroke and evaluated the effects of time since stroke, spasticity, and motor recovery on the body composition specifically within the first year after stroke found lean tissue mass and bone mineral content of the paretic side to be significantly lower than those of the non affected side; a significant correlation was found between the lean tissue mass and bone mineral content of both the paretic and non affected legs after adjusting for age and weight. On the contrary bone mineral content and lean tissue mass of both the paretic and non affected sides were negatively correlated with time since stroke in patients with stroke for less than 1 year and a higher lean tissue mass and bone mineral content were found in patients with moderate to high spasticity in comparison with patients with low or no spasticity (Celik et al., 2008).

3.4 Cerebral palsy

Bone mineralization in children with CP has been found lower (bone-mineral values for the total body and total proximal femur) than sex- and age-matched able bodied children. This is illustrated by the BMC Z - scores determined at each skeletal site. The factors that contribute to low bone mineralization include genetic, hormonal, and nutritional problems (especially calcium and vitamin D) and weight-bearing physical activity, oral-motor dysfunction and anticonvulsant medication (Henderson et al., 1995).

Free fat mass (FFM) in cerebral palsy subjects was found significantly lower than that in a normal adolescent population. In 60% of the studied population body fat exceeded the 90th

percentile for age, even if most of the CP children had a low height and weight for age. In female subjects anthropometric measurements were highly correlated with measures of body fatness. Measuring fat by ^{18}O dilution a hydration factor of 0.73 was assumed for FFM. A possible increase in the hydration factor would diminish measured FFM meaning that body fat appears increased. Moreover muscle spasms and spasticity in CP subjects deplete body glycogen. If glycogen is reduced the intracellular water would be reduced and the ratio extracellular water/total body water would increase. The same could result with a loss of body cell mass or an increase in the hydration factor (Bandini et al., 1991).

4. Conclusions

Other important issues according alterations of body composition are the completeness of lesions (an absence of sensory or motor function below the neurological level, including the lowest sacral segment), because body composition seems to be worst than subjects with incomplete lesions (partial preservation of motor and/or sensory function below the neurological level, including the lowest sacral segment) (Sabo et al., 1991; Demirel et al., 1998; Garland et al., 1992) and aging which contributes to major alterations of body composition.

In disabled subjects the most important issue according to body composition is how to promote optimal body weight to reduce risk of diseases such as coronary heart disease, non-insulin dependent diabetes mellitus, lipid abnormalities and fractures because of bone loss. Dietary changes, individualized physical activity programs and medication should be taken in mind in therapy when we deal with this subgroup of subjects. However, self-management of dietary changes to improve weight control and disease should be the case, which means they need to follow diets with lower energy intake and at the same time to eat regularly foods rich in nutrients (Groah et al., 2009).

We need to take in mind that healthy BMI values often underestimate body fat and may mask the adiposity and spasticity did not defend skeletal muscle mass and bone, supporting the concept that in neurologic disabilities the myopathic muscle could not recognize correctly the stimulation because of the neurogenic injury. Moreover, disabled subjects mostly transfer much of the weight-bearing demands of daily activities to their upper extremities reducing the weight-bearing of the affected paralyzed muscles triggering a cycle of added muscle atrophy which interacts with the continuous catabolic action caused by the neurogenic factor. Finally, an irreversible (once established) decline in bone mineral density, bone mineral content as well as geometric characteristics of bone is expected and the duration of lesion-injury is positively correlated with the degree of bone loss.

Further research about body composition is needed in all physical disabilities and more longitudinal studies to quantitate and monitor body composition changes and to modify our therapeutic interventions. However, prevention rather than treatment may have the greatest potential to alleviate these major complications. Therapies should focus on how to perform weight bearing, standing or therapeutically walking activities early in the rehabilitation program to gain benefits according to muscles and bones.

5. References

Bandini LG, Schoeller DA, Fukagawa NK, Wykes LJ, Dietz WH. Body composition and energy expenditure in adolescents with cerebral palsy or myelodysplasia.Pediatr Res. 1991 Jan;29(1):70-7.

Bauman WA, Spungen AM, Raza M, Rothstein J, Zhang RL, Zhong YG, Tsuruta M, Shahidi R, Pierson RN Jr, Wang J, et al. Coronary artery disease: metabolic risk factors and latent disease in individuals with paraplegia. Mt Sinai J Med. 1992 Mar;59(2):163-8.

Bauman WA, Spungen AM, Zhong YG, Mobbs CV. Plasma leptin is directly related to body adiposity in subjects with spinal cord injury. Horm Metab Res. 1996;28:732-6.

Bauman WA, Spungen AM. 1994 Disorders of carbohydrate and lipid metabolism in veterans with paraplegia or quadriplegia: A model of premature aging. Metabolism .43: 749.756.

Bender R, Trautner C, Spraul M, Berger M. Assessment of excess mortality in obesity. Am J Epidemiol. 1998;147:42-8.

Biering-Sorensen F, Bohr HH, Schaadt OP. Longitudinal study of bone mineral content in the lumbar spine, the forearm and the lower extremities after spinal cord injury. Eur J Clin Invest. 1990; 20:330-5.

Buchholz AC, Bugaresti JM. A review of body mass index and waist circumference as markers of obesity and coronary heart disease risk in persons with chronic spinal cord injury. Spinal Cord. 2005;43:513-8.

Castro MJ, Apple DF Jr, Hillegass EA, and Dudley GA. Influence of complete spinal cord injury on skeletal muscle cross-sectional area within the first 6 months of injury. Eur J Appl Physiol 80: 373–378, 1999a.

Castro MJ, Apple DF Jr, Staron RS, Campos GE, Dudley GA. Influence of complete spinal cord injury on skeletal muscle within 6 mo of injury. J Appl Physiol. 1999b;86:350-8.

Celik B, Ones K, Ince N. Body composition after stroke. Int J Rehabil Res. 2008 Mar;31(1):93-6.

Chad KE, McKay HA, Zello GA, Bailey DA, Faulkner RA, Snyder RE. Body composition in nutritionally adequate ambulatory and non-ambulatory children with cerebral palsy and a healthy reference group. Dev Med Child Neurol. 2000 May;42(5):334-9.

Chantraine A, Nusgens B, Lapiere CM. Bone remodelling during the development of osteoporosis in paraplegia. Calcif Tissue Int. 1986;38:323-7.

Chow YW, Inman C, Pollintine P, Sharp CA, Haddaway MJ, el Masry W, Davie MW.Ultrasound bone densitometry and dual energy X-ray absorptiometry in patients with spinal cord injury: a cross-sectional study. Spinal Cord. 1996 Dec;34(12):736-41.

Clarys JP, Martin AD, Drinkwater DT. Gross tissue weights in the human body by cadaver dissection. Hum Biol. 1984;56:459-73.

Clasey JL, Janowiak AL, Gater DR Relationship between regional bone density measurements and the time since injury in adults with spinal cord injuries. Arch Phys Med Rehabil. 2004;85:59–64

Correia ML, Morgan DA, Mitchell JL, Sivitz WI, Mark AL, Haynes WG. Role of corticotrophin-releasing factor in effects of leptin on sympathetic nerve activity and arterial pressure. Hypertension. 2001;38:384-8.

Coupaud S, McLean AN, Allan DB. Role of peripheral quantitative computed tomography in identifying disuse osteoporosis in paraplegia. Skeletal Radiol. 2009 Oct;38(10):989-95.

Dauty M, Perrouin Verbe B, Maugars Y, Dubois C, Mathe JF. Supralesional and sublesional bone mineral density in spinal cord-injured patients. Bone. 2000;27:305-9.

Demirel G, Yilmaz H, Paker N, Onel S. Osteoporosis after spinal cord injury. Spinal Cord. 1998;36:8

Dionyssiotis Y, Lyritis GP, Papaioannou N, Papagelopoulos P, Thomaides T. Influence of neurological level of injury in bones, muscles, and fat in paraplegia. J Rehabil Res Dev. 2009;46(8):1037-44.

Dionyssiotis Y, Trovas G, Galanos A, Raptou P, Papaioannou N, Papagelopoulos P, Petropoulou K, Lyritis GP. Bone loss and mechanical properties of tibia in spinal cord injured men. J Musculoskelet Neuronal Interact. 2007 Jan-Mar;7(1):62-8.

Dionyssiotis Y. (2011d). Bone Loss in Spinal Cord Injury and Multiple Sclerosis. In: JH Stone, M Blouin, editors. International Encyclopedia of Rehabilitation, av. online: http://cirrie.buffalo.edu/encyclopedia/en/article/340/

Dionyssiotis Y. Changes in bone density and strength of the tibia and alterations of lean and fat mass in chronic paraplegic men. Doctoral Dissertation Laboratory for Research of the Musculoskeletal System, University of Athens, Athens, 2008a.

Dionyssiotis Y, Petropoulou K, Rapidi CA, Papagelopoulos PJ, Papaioannou N, Galanos A, Papadaki P, and Lyritis GP. Body Composition in Paraplegic Men. Journal of Clinical Densitometry. 2008b;11: 437-43.

Dionyssiotis, Y. Bone loss and fractures in multiple sclerosis: focus on epidemiologic and physiopathological features. Int J Gen Med. 2011b; 4: 505-9.

Dionyssiotis, Y. Spinal cord injury-related bone impairment and fractures: an update on epidemiology and physiopathological mechanisms. J Musculoskelet Neuronal Interact. 2011c; 11(3):257-65.

Dionyssiotis, Y, Lyritis GP, Mavrogenis AF, Papagelopoulos PJ. Factors influencing bone loss in paraplegia. Hippokratia. 2011a ; 15(1):54-9.

Elias CF, Lee C, Kelly J, Aschkenasi C, Ahima RS, Couceyro PR, Kuhar MJ, Saper CB, Elmquist JK. Leptin activates hypothalamic CART neurons projecting to the spinal cord. Neuron. 1998;21:1375-85.

Ferretti J.L., Cointry G.R., Capozza R.F., Zanchetta J.R. Dual energy X-ray absorptiometry. Skeletal Muscle: Pathology, Diagnosis and Management of Disease. V.R.Preedy, T.J.Peters (eds),Greenwich Medical Media, Ltd., London, 2001; p.451-458.

Forbes GB, Simon W, Amatruda JM. Is bioimpedance a good predictor of body-composition change? Am J Clin Nutr 1992;56:4-6.

Forbes GB. Human body composition: growth, aging, nutrition, and activity. New York: Springer-Verlag; 1987.

Formica CA, Cosman F, Nieves J, Herbert J, Lindsay R. Reduced bone mass and fat-free mass in women with multiple sclerosis: effects of ambulatory status and glucocorticoid Use. Calcif Tissue Int. 1997 Aug;61(2):129-33.

Frey-Rindova P, de Bruin ED, Stussi E, Dambacher MA, Dietz V. Bone mineral density in upper and lower extremities during 12 months after spinal cord injury measured by peripheral quantitative computed tomography. Spinal Cord. 2000;38:26–32.

Frisancho RA. New norms of upper limb fat and muscle areas for assessment of nutritional status. Am J Clin Nutr 1981;34:2540–2545.

Fruhbeck G, Jebb SA, Prentice AM. Leptin: physiology and pathophysiology. Clin Physiol. 1998;18:399-419.

Garland DE, Stewart CA, Adkins RH, Hu SS, Rosen C, Liotta FJ, Weinstein DA. 1992. Osteoporosis after spinal cord injury. J Orthop Res .10 :371.378.

Gorgey AS, Dudley GA. Skeletal muscle atrophy and increased intramuscular fat after incomplete spinal cord injury. Spinal Cord 2007;45(4):304–309.

Groah SL, Nash MS, Ljungberg IH, Libin A, Hamm LF, Ward E, Burns PA, Enfield G. Nutrient intake and body habitus after spinal cord injury: an analysis by sex and level of injury. J Spinal Cord Med. 2009;32:25-33.

Hafer-Macko CE, Ryan AS, Ivey FM, Macko RF. Skeletal muscle changes after hemiparetic stroke and potential beneficial effects of exercise intervention strategies. J Rehabil Res Dev. 2008;45(2):261-72.

Haque MS, Minokoshi Y, Hamai M, Iwai M, Horiuchi M, Shimazu T. Role of the sympathetic nervous system and insulin in enhancing glucose uptake in peripheral tissues after intrahypothalamic injection of leptin in rats. Diabetes. 1999;48:1706-12.

Henderson RC, Lin PP, Greene WB. (1995). Bone-mineral density in children and adolescents who have spastic cerebral palsy.*Journal of Bone and Joint Surgery* 77A: 1671–81.

Heymsfield SB, Wang J, Heshka S, Kehayias JJ, Pierson RN. Dual-photon absorptiometry: comparison of bone mineral and soft tissue mass measurements in vivo with established methods. Am J Clin Nutr. 1989 Jun;49(6):1283-9.

Hildreth HG, Johnson RK, Goran MI, Contompasis SH. Body composition in adults with cerebral palsy by dual-energy X-ray absorptiometry, bioelectrical impedance analysis, and skinfold anthropometry compared with the 18O isotope-dilution technique. Am J Clin Nutr. 1997 Dec;66(6):1436-42.

Horowitz JF, Coppack SW, Paramore D, Cryer PE, Zhao G, Klein S. Effect of short-term fasting on lipid kinetics in lean and obese women. Am J Physiol. 1999;276:E278-84.

Horowitz JF, Klein S. Whole body and abdominal lipolytic sensitivity to epinephrine is suppressed in upper body obese women. Am J Physiol Endocrinol Metab. 2000;278:E1144-52.

Ingemann-Hansen T, Halkjaer-Kristensen J. Lean and fat component of the human thigh: the effects of immobilization in plaster and subsequent physical training. *Scand J Rehabil Med.* 1977;9:67–72

Jeon JY, Steadward RD, Wheeler GD, Bell G, McCargar L, Harber V. Intact sympathetic nervous system is required for leptin effects on resting metabolic rate in people with spinal cord injury. J Clin Endocrinol Metab. 2003;88:402-7.

Jiang SD, Dai LY, Jiang LS. Osteoporosis after spinal cord injury. Osteoporos Int. 2006;17:180-92.

Jones LM, Goulding A, Gerrard DF. DEXA: a practical and accurate tool to demonstrate total and regional bone loss, lean tissue loss and fat mass gain in paraplegia. Spinal Cord. 1998;36:637-40

Kent-Braun JA, Ng AV, Castro M, et al. Strength, skeletal muscle composition and enzyme activity in multiple sclerosis. J Appl Physiol 1997;83:1998-2004.

Kent-Braun JA, Sharma KR, Weiner MW, Miller RG. Effects of exercise on muscle activation and metabolism in multiple sclerosis.Muscle Nerve 1994;17:1162-9.

Kocina P. Body composition of spinal cord injured adults. Sports Medicine. 1997; 23:48-60.

Krassioukov AV, Bunge RP, Pucket WR, Bygrave MA. The changes in human spinal sympathetic preganglionic neurons after spinal cord injury. Spinal Cord. 1999;37:6-13.

Krupp, LB, Serafin DJ, Christodoulou C. Multiple sclerosis-associated fatigue. Expert Rev Neurother. 2010;10:1437-47.

Kunkel CF, Scremin AM, Eisenberg B, Garcia JF, Roberts S, Martinez S. Effect of "standing" on spasticity, contracture, and osteoporosis in paralyzed males. Arch Phys Med Rehabil. 1993;74:73–8.

Kuperminc MN, Stevenson RD. Growth and nutrition disorders in children with cerebral palsy. Dev Disabil Res Rev. 2008;14(2):137-46.

LaForgia J, Dollman J, Dale MJ, Withers RT, Hill AM. Validation of DXA body composition estimates in obese men and women. Obesity (Silver Spring). 2009;17:821-6.

Lambert CP, Archer RL, Evans WJ. Body composition in ambulatory women with multiple sclerosis. Arch Phys Med Rehabil 2002;83:1559-61.

Laskey MA. Dual-energy X-ray absorptiometry and body composition. Nutrition.1996 Jan;12(1):45-51.

Lazo MG, Shirazi P, Sam M, Giobbie-Hurder A, Blacconiere MJ, Muppidi M. Osteoporosis and risk of fracture in men with spinal cord injury. Spinal Cord. 2001;39:208-14.

Leslie WD, Nance PW. Dissociated hip and spine demineralization: a specific finding in spinal cord injury. Arch Phys Med Rehabil. 1993; 74:960-4.

Liu LF, Roberts R, Moyer-Mileur L, Samson-Fang L. Determination of body composition in children with cerebral palsy: bioelectrical impedance analysis and anthropometry vs dual-energy x-ray absorptiometry. J Am Diet Assoc. 2005 May;105(5):794-7.

Lohman TG. Applicability of body composition techniques and constants for children and youth. In: Pandolf KB, editor. Exercise and sport sciences reviews. Vol 14. New York: Macmillan; 1986. p 325-57.

Lohman, TG.; Roche, AF.; Martorell, R. Anthropometric standardization reference manual. Human Kinetics Books; Champaign: 1988

Maffei M, Halaas J, Ravussin E, Pratley RE, Lee GH, Zhang Y, Fei H, Kim S, Lallone R, Ranganathan S, et al. Leptin levels in human and rodent: measurement of plasma leptin and ob RNA in obese and weight-reduced subjects. Nat Med. 1995;1:1155-61.

Mahon AK, Flynn MG, Iglay HB, Stewart LK, Johnson CA, McFarlin BK, Campbell WW. Measurement of body composition changes with weight loss in postmenopausal women: comparison of methods. J Nutr Health Aging. 2007;11:203-13.

Maimoun L, Fattal C, Micallef JP, Peruchon E, Rabischong P. Bone loss in spinal cord-injured patients: from physiopathology to therapy. Spinal Cord. 2006;44:203-10.

McDonald CM, Abresch-Meyer AL, Nelson MD, Widman LM. Body mass index and body composition measures by dual x-ray absorptiometry in patients aged 10 to 21 years with spinal cord injury. J Spinal Cord Med. 2007;30:S97-104.

Mitsiopoulos N, Baumgartner RN, Heymsfield SB, Lyons W, Gallagher D, and Ross R. Cadaver validation of skeletal muscle measurement by magnetic resonance imaging and computerized tomography. J Appl Physiol. 85: 115–122, 1998.

Modlesky CM, Bickel CS, Slade JM, Meyer RA, Cureton KJ, Dudley GA. Assessment of skeletal muscle mass in men with spinal cord injury using dual-energy X-ray absorptiometry and magnetic resonance imaging. J Appl Physiol. 2004;96:561-5.

Mojtahedi MC, Valentine RJ, Arngrímsson SA, Wilund KR, Evans EM. The association between regional body composition and metabolic outcomes in athletes with spinal cord injury. Spinal Cord. 2008 Mar;46:192-7.

National Institutes of Health Technology Assessment Conference Statement. Bioelectrical impedance analysis in body composition measurement. Bethesda, MD: National Institutes of Health, 1994:12-4

Ng AV, Kent-Braun JA. Quantitation of lower physical activity in persons with multiple sclerosis. Med Sci Sports Exerc 1997;29: 517-23.

Ogilvie C, Bowker P, Rowley DI. The physiological benefits of paraplegic orthotically aided walking. Paraplegia. 1993;31:111-5.

Olgiati R, Burgunder JM, Mumenthaler M. Increased energy cost of walking in multiple sclerosis: effect of spasticity, ataxia, and weakness. Arch Phys Med Rehabil 1988;69:846-9.

Olle MM, Pivarnik JM, Klish WJ, Morrow JR Jr. Body composition of sedentary and physically active spinal cord injured individuals estimated from total body electrical conductivity. Arch Phys Med Rehabil. 1993;74:706-10.

Patrick J, Gisel E. Nutrition for the feeding impaired child. J Neuro Rehab 1990;4:115–119.

Peppler WW, Mazess RB. 1981. Total body bone mineral and lean body mass by dual-photon absorptiometry. Calcif Tissue Int 33:353-359

Pietrobelli A, Formica C, Wang AM, Heymsfield SB. 1996. Dual-energy X-ray absorptiometry body composition model: review of physical concepts. Am J Physiol 271 (Endocrinol Metab 34): E941-E951

Rittweger J, Beller G, Ehrig J, Jung C, Koch U, Ramolla J, Schmidt F, Newitt D, Majumdar S, Schiessl H, Felsenberg D. Bone-muscle strength indices for the human lower leg. Bone. 2000;27:319-26.

Ryan AS, Dobrovolny CL, Silver KH, Smith GV, Macko RF. Cardiovascular fitness after stroke: Role of muscle mass and gait deficit severity. J Stroke Cerebro Dis 2000;9:185–191.

Ryan AS, Dobrovolny CL, Smith GV, Silver KH, Macko RF. Hemiparetic muscle atrophy and increased intramuscular fat in stroke patients. Arch Phys Med Rehabil 2002;83(12):1703–1707.

Sabo D, Blaich S, Wenz W, Hohmann M, Loew M, Gerner HJ. Osteoporosis in patients with paralysis after spinal cord injury: a cross sectional study in 46 male patients with dual-energy X-ray absorptiometry. Arch Orthop Trauma Surg. 2001;121:75–8.

Samson-Fang LJ, Stevenson RD. Identification of malnutrition in children with cerebral palsy: poor performance of weight-for-height centiles. Dev Med Child Neurol. 2000;42:162–168

Scelsi R. Skeletal muscle pathology after spinal cord injury. Basic Appl Myol. 2001;11:75-85.

Schonheyder F, Heilskov NCS, Olesen K. Isotopic studies on the mechanism of negative nitrogen balance produced by immobilization. Scand Clin Lab Invest.1954;6:178-188.

Seidell JC, Verschuren WM, van Leer EM, Kromhout D. Overweight, underweight, and mortality. A prospective study of 48.287 men and women. Arch Intern Med. 1996;156:958-63.

Shields RK, Dudley-Javoroski S. Musculoskeletal adaptations in chronic spinal cord injury: effects of long-term soleus electrical stimulation training. Neurorehabil Neural Repair. 2007;21:169-79.

Shields RK. Muscular, skeletal, and neural adaptations following spinal cord injury. J Orthop Sports Phys Ther. 2002;32:65-74.

Sioka C, Fotopoulos A, Georgiou A, Papakonstantinou S, Pelidou SH, Kyritsis AP, Kalef-Ezra JA. Body composition in ambulatory patients with multiple sclerosis. J Clin Densitom. 2011 Aug 9.

Slaughter MH, Lohman TG, Boileau RA, et al. Skinfold equations for estimation of body fatness in children and youth. Hum Biol 1988;60:709–723.

Smeltzer SC, Zimmerman V, Capriotti T. Osteoporosis risk and low bone mineral density in women with physical disabilities. Arch Phys Med Rehabil. 2005;86:582-6.

Spungen AM, Adkins RH, Stewart CA, Wang J, Pierson RN Jr, Waters RL, Bauman WA. Factors influencing body composition in persons with spinal cord injury: a cross-sectional study. J Appl Physiol. 2003;95: 2398–2407.

Stallings VA, Cronk CE, Zemel BS, Charney EB. Body composition in children with spastic quadriplegic cerebral palsy. J Pediatr. 1995 May;126(5 Pt 1):833-9.

Steen B, Lundgren BK, Isaksson B. Body composition at age 70, 75, 79, and 81 years: a longitudinal population study. In: Chandra RK, ed. Nutrition, Immunity and Illness in the Elderly. New York, NY: Pergamon Press, Inc; 1985:49-52.

Stevenson RD, Roberts CD, Vogtle L. The effects of non-nutritional factors on growth in cerebral palsy. Dev Med Child Neurol. 1995;37: 124–130

Szollar SM, Martin EM, Parthemore JG, Sartoris DJ, Deftos LJ. Densitometric patterns of spinal cord injury associated bone loss. Spinal Cord. 1997 Jun;35(6):374-82.

Tsuzuku S, Ikegami Y, Yabe K. Bone mineral density differences between paraplegic and quadriplegic patients: a cross-sectional study. Spinal Cord. 1999; 37:358-61.

Uebelhart D, Demiaux-Domenech B, Roth M, Chantraine A. Bone metabolism in spinal cord injured individuals and in others who have prolonged immobilisation. A review. Paraplegia 1995; 33: 669-673.

Unosson M, Ek AC, Bjurulf P, von Schenck H, Larsson J. Feeding dependence and nutritional status after acute stroke. Stroke 1994, 25(2):366-371.

Van Der Ploeg GE, Withers RT, Laforgia J. Percent body fat via DEXA: comparison with a four-compartment model. J Appl Physiol. 2003;94:499-506.

Wang YH, Huang TS, Liang HW, Su TC, Chen SY, Wang TD. Fasting serum levels of adiponectin, ghrelin, and leptin in men with spinal cord injury. Arch Phys Med Rehabil. 2005;86:1964-8.

Part 3

Miscellaneous

7

Internal Design of the Dry Human Ulna by DXA

S. Aguado-Henche, A. Bosch-Martín,
P. Spottorno-Rubio and R. Rodríguez-Torres
University of Alcalá
Spain

1. Introduction

Dual energy X-ray absorptiometry (DXA) has been used to study dry bones such as spine, femur, jaw... to detect the first onsets of the ossification centers; In clinical practice, DXA is widely used for diagnosis and evaluation of osteoporosis, and a new generation of DXA scanners offers software for performing vertebral morphometry analysis (Blake & Fogelman, 1997). Also, many bone analyses have been performed on experimental animals using DXA (Tsujio et al., 2009).

Studies on the spatial distribution of bone mineral density (BMD) in the whole bone, reflecting its morphological pattern are scarce (Gómez-Pellico et al., 1993 & Fernández-Camacho et al., 1996). In addition, there are just few studies regarding the anthropometric characteristics of the human ulna (Weber et al., 2009).

In order to improve the treatment of the elbow's injury, knowledge related to the resistance of the bone is important to understand the origin of the fractures as well as to improve elbow fracture recovery (Heep, 2007). Most studies investigate the humeral component, while the ulna component is not being studied as much (Goto, 2009).

In order to develop an implant that carries out the mechanical characteristics of a native bone, we must study the trabecular architecture of the human ulna proximal extremity.

1.1 Brief anatomy of the human ulna

The ulna is a long bone, placed at the medial side of the forearm, parallel to the radius. It is divisible into a body and two extremities. Its upper extremity, of great thickness and strength, forms a large part of the elbow-joint; the bone diminishes in size from above downward, its lower extremity being very small, and excluded from the wrist-joint by the interposition of an articular disk (the ulna articulates with the humerus and radius).

The upper extremity presents two curved processes, the olecranon and the coronoid process; and two concave, articular cavities, the trochlear and radial notches. The olecranon is a large, thick, curved eminence, situated at the upper and back part of the ulna. The coronoid process is a triangular eminence projecting forward from the upper and front part of the ulna. Its base is continuous with the body of the bone, and of considerable strength.

Its antero-inferior surface is concave, and marked by a rough impression for the insertion of the brachialis muscle. The trochlear notch is a large depression, formed by the olecranon and the coronoid process, and serving for articulation with the trochlea of the humerus. The notch is concave from above downward, and divided into a medial and a lateral portion by a smooth ridge running from the summit of the olecranon to the tip of the coronoid process. The radial notch is a narrow, oblong, articular depression on the lateral side of the coronoid process; it receives the circumferential articular surface of the head of the radius. The lower extremity of the ulna is small, and presents two eminences; the lateral and larger is a rounded, articular eminence, termed the head of the ulna; the medial, narrower and more projecting is a non-articular eminence named the styloid process.

The ulna is ossified from three centers: one for the body, the inferior extremity, and the top of the olecranon. Ossification begins about the eighth week of fetal life. About the fourth year, a center appears in the middle of the ulnar head, and soon extends into the styloid process. About the tenth year, a center appears in the olecranon near its extremity. The upper epiphysis joins the body about the sixteenth year and the lower about the twentieth.

2. Objective

In this chapter, we set out to show, by means of densitometric analysis with dual energy X-ray absorptiometry (DXA) the internal design of the human ulna, to verify that the bone tissue distribution is not homogeneous and that this corresponds to the trabecular architecture of the bone.

3. Material and method

A random sample of 41 dry right ulnas from the skeletal collection of the Anatomy and Embriology Department of the University of Alcala was studied excluding those bones which presented any alterations or damage. A Norland XR-26 densitometer, software 2.5 (Norland Co., Fort Atkinson, WI, USA; Emsor SA, Madrid) was used for all studies. Each scan session was preceded by a calibration routine using a standard calibration block supplied by the manufacturer.

The bone is placed well centred on the examining board. It is important to check for stability so as not to vary its position during the study. Cotton gauze may be needed for an optimal stabilization. The bones are exposed directly, without any water or other materials that may resemble soft tissue.

For the densitometric analysis of the human ulna structure two projections were performed: lateral and antero-posterior.

For the study in two positions, the reference will be the ridge of the trochlear notch of the epiphyseal ulna (incisura trochlearis) which corresponds to the throat of the trochlea -humerus- (Gómez-Oliveros, 1962).

- Anteroposterior Position: The axis of the ridge of the trochlear notch is perpendicular to the axis of the examining board.
- Lateral Position: The axis of the ridge of the trochlear notch is parallel to the axis of the examining board.

To begin the scan, (figure 1) the starting point was placed 0, 5 cm directly above the upper extremity. A baseline point was marked under the lower extremity. A third point (goal line) was marked 1 cm from the more lateral part of the bone.

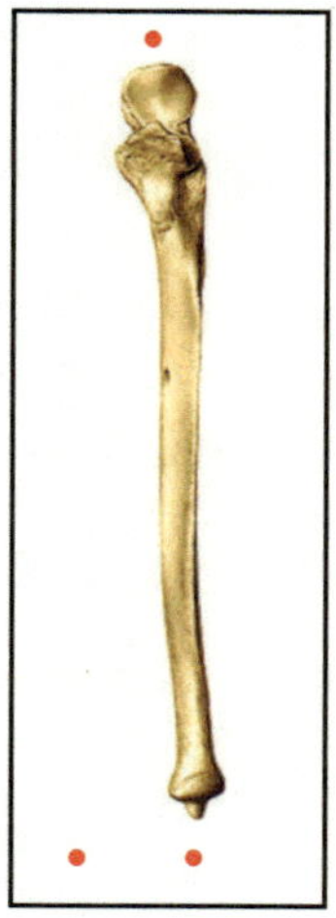

Fig. 1. Definition of the exploration area

This technique has high accuracy and precision, approaching 1%. The speed of scanning was 60 mms, with an interlinear space of 1 mm and point by point resolution of 1 mm horizontal x 1 mm vertical. The defined exploration was completed as outlined in an average time of 10-15 min. Scan acquisition and scan analyses were performed by one investigator (figure 2).

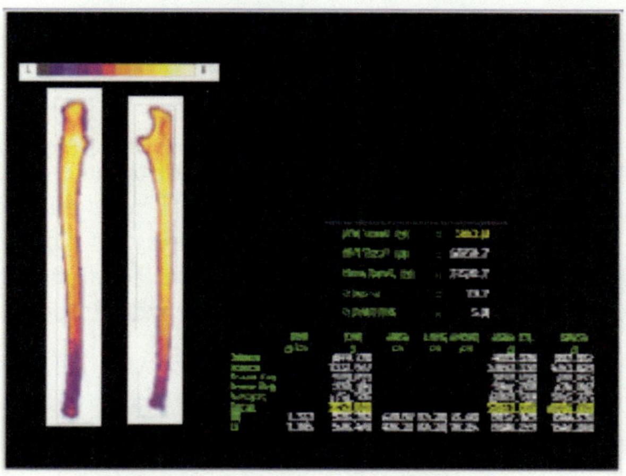

Fig. 2. Densitometric image of the ulna.

Dry ulna calculations were performed for the following magnitudes:

BMD: Bone mineral density, in grams / cm^2.

BMC: Bone mineral content, in grams. BMC is defined as the mass of mineral contained in an entire bone or as the mass of mineral per unit bone length. Bone mineral content is obviously a size-dependent parameter (Schoenau, 2004).

AREA: Measured area, in square centimetres (cm^2).
LENGTH: Total length of the bone, in centimetres (cm).
WIDTH: Total width of the bone, in centimetres (cm).

For the purpose of this survey, in both projections five equal regions of interest (ROI) were selected: proximal (ROI-1), proximal-intermediate (ROI-2), intermediate (ROI-3), distal-intermediate (ROI-4) and distal (ROI-5). The total region corresponded to the area of the full length and height of the bone (figure 3).

All statistical calculations were performed using Statgraphics Plus (version 5.1) and SPSS (Statistical Package for Social Sciences), version 15.0. The means and standard deviation (SD) for bone mineral density (BMD) and bone mineral content (BMC) were calculated. The bone densities and the bone contents of the various regions of the ulna in the 2 projections were compared by Student's *t* test for paired samples.

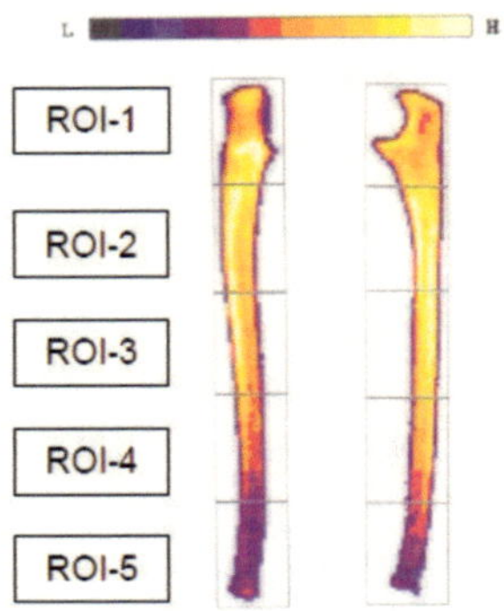

Fig. 3. Regions of interest.

4. Results

DXA indicates that the higher BMD is in the proximal-intermediate region (R2), which is the part of the ulna that bears the higher force of traction. The higher BMC is found in the proximal region (R1) which corresponds to the coronoid process. Lower BMD and BMC are found in the distal region (R5). The total BMD shows significant statistical differences ($p \leq 0.001$), which indicates the heterogeneous nature of the distribution of bone mass in the studied bone.

In tables 1 - 4 we present the statistic descriptions of the densitometry variables studied in both.

Projection A-P	Mínimum	Máximum	Mean	SD
Total BMD	0,40	0,97	0,69	0,14
Total BMC	13,10	46,40	28,75	8,63
Total Area	30,73	51,54	41,05	5,70
Total Lenght	20,40	27,90	24,51	1,66
Total Width	2,55	4,35	3,35	0,40

Table 1. Descriptive statistics of the total ulna in projection antero-posterior (n=41). SD: Standard deviation.

Projection LAT	Mínimum	Máximum	Mean	SD
Total BMD	0,38	0,94	0,67	0,14
Total BMC	13,15	46,74	28,72	8,50
Total Area	32,81	52,51	41,84	5,25
Total Lenght	20,40	28,05	24,50	1,66
Total Width	3,15	6,60	4,08	0,59

Table 2. Descriptive statistics of the total ulna in projection lateral (n=41). SD: Standard deviation.

	ROI 1		ROI 2		ROI 3		ROI 4		ROI 5	
	Media	SD	Media	SD	Media	SD	Media	SD	Media	SD
AP-Area	10,58	1,57	9,08	1,33	8,12	1,42	7,02	1,01	6,22	0,94
AP-Lenght	4,88	0,33	4,88	0,33	5,03	0,41	4,88	0,33	4,88	0,33
LAT-Area	11,68	1,52	8,94	1,24	8,09	1,07	6,98	0,82	6,24	1,00
LAT-Lenght	4,88	0,33	4,88	0,33	5,03	0,43	4,88	0,33	4,88	0,33

Table 3. Descriptive statistics of the regions of interest in projections antero-posterior (AP) and lateral (LAT). n=41. SD: Standard deviation.

ANTERO-POSTERIOR VIEW BMD	ANTERO-POSTERIOR VIEW BMC		LATERAL VIEW BMD	LATERAL VIEW BMC
0,754	8,136	ROI-1	0,678	8,07
0,81	7,513	ROI-2	0,819	7,442
0,734	6,089	ROI-3	0,750	6,169
0,599	4,289	ROI-4	0,608	4,297
0,447	2,814	ROI-5	0,453	2,819
ULNA TOTAL BMD 0,69			ULNA TOTAL BMD 0,67	
ULNA TOTAL BMC 28,75			ULNA TOTAL BMC 28,72	

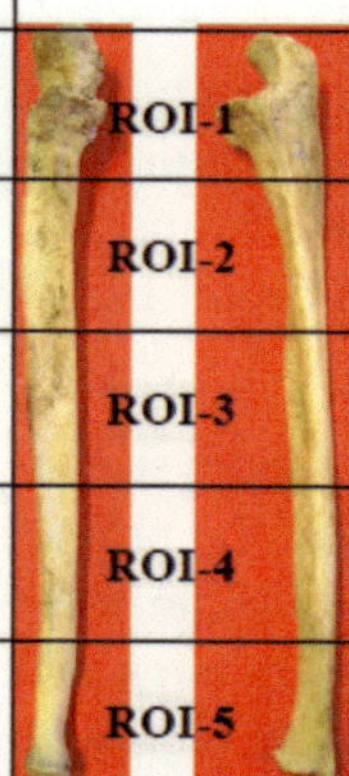

Table 4. BMD (in grams/cm^2) and BMC (in grams) of the regions of interest.

5. Discussion

Dual energy X-ray absorptiometry (DXA) allows us to gather quantitative information on bone mineral content (BMC) and bone mineral density (BMD) of the bone (Wahner et al., 1985). As previously reported (Hvid et al., 1985), there is a close relationship between bone mass and bone strength.

In literature, there are various studies on long bones, such as the femur, the tibia, the humerus and the radius (Wahner et al., 1985; Kawashima & Uhthoff, 1991; Gómez-Pellico et al., 1993; D'Amelio et al., 2002) but we haven't found any references that study the distribution of the BMD in the ulna that describes it´s construction systematics .

According to Wolf's law (Viladot , 2001), the bone adapts its size, shape and structure to the mechanical requirements it receives. Furthermore, Pauwels (Pauwels, 1980; Miralles, 1998) suggests that the mass of the cortical bone is distributed along its axis proportionally to the amount of tensions it receives. In our analysis, we find a wider BMD in the intermediate-proximal region (ROI-2), which corresponds to the region of the bone exposed to the mechanical flexions and to the transmission of weight charges while the superior member is in the extended position. Three different soft tissue structures insert in or attach to the coronoid process, the articular capsule, the tendon of the brachialis muscle, and the anterior band of the ulnar collateral ligament (Fowler & Chung, 2006). Furthermore, the transmission of weight charges travels through the coronoid apophysis, situated in the proximal region, which present the wider BMC in both projections, however, DXA is unable to distinguish between cortical and trabecular bone (Griffith & Genant, 2008).

This and other similar studies will contribute to a better understanding of stress related fractures which are quite scarce in the ulna and cannot easily be found in literature (Chen, WC et al., 1991). Most fractures occur in the middle third of the diaphysis and surrounding areas as a result of mechanical stressing forces of the forearm in a specific position, especially in athletes (Rettig, 1983).

Some authors have agreed on the homogeneous nature of the different diaphysarial regions of the long bones that they study (femur, humerus and tibia) (Gómez Pellico et al., 1993; Fernández-Camacho et al., 1996). As far as the ulna is concerned, BMD displays a more heterogeneous distribution, since we find statistical differences in all studied regions and on the entire bone.

In studies of the dry femur with DXA, epiphysiary regions are those with less BMD which, added to the mechanical requirements of the physiology of the articulation, would explain how hip ostheoporotic fractures occur (Gómez-Pellico et al., 1993). Furthermore, most studies with DXA are based on BMD variations related to loss of bone mass of pathologic nature (McCarthy et al., 1991). This also happens with "in vivo" studies of the radius. Due to the high rate fractures of the distal radius in children, the use this bone to measure BMD, is increasing, essentially as thus to predict the risk of fracture (Kalkwarf et al., 2011). The study of the dry radius with DXA would define its construction systematics.

The results obtained with the DXA technique showed that BMD agrees with the arrangement of the trabecular system in the human ulna, previously described by some authors (Testut & Latarjet, 1949; Gómez-Oliveros, 1962).

In addition, fractures of the coronoid process are rarely seen as an isolated injury. They are encountered more frecuently in association with radial head fractures (Weber et al., 2009).

Due to frequent complications associated with reconstructive surgery for the elbow, implant loosening, periprosthetic fracture, implant failure... (Kim, 2011), that remains higher than arthroplasty of other joints (Sanchez-Sotelo, 2011), the findings that result from this study could contribute to the improvement of elbow prosthesis.

6. Conclusions

The human ulna presents a heterogeneous distribution of the BMD. This study confirms that the higher mechanical requirements in the ulna are in the proximal extremity. The differences found in the ulna BMD allows us a better understanding of the construction systematics and their functional activity. We conclude that bone densitometry, measured by the DXA technique, is useful for assessing trabecular architecture of the human skeleton. This study may provide some useful information on plate application for the treatment of the elbow injuries.

7. References

Blake, GM. & Fogelman I. (1997). Technical principles, *Seminars in Nuclear Medicine* 27(3):210-228.

D'Amelio, P., Panattoni, GL. & Isaia GC. (2002). Densitometric study of human developing dry bones: a review, *Journal of Clinical Densitometric* 5(1):73-78.

Chen, WC., Hsu, WY & Wu, JJ (1991). Stress fracture of the diaphysis of the ulna, *International Orthopaedics* 15: 197-198.

Fernández Camacho, FJ., Morante Martínez, P., Rodríguez Torres, R., Cortés García, A. & Gómez Pellico, L. (1996). Densitometric analysis of the human calcaneus, *Journal of Anatomy* 189:205-209.

Fowler, K. & Chung, C. (2006). Normal MR imaging anatomy of the elbow, *Radiologic Clinics of North America* 44(4):553-567.

Gómez Pellico, L., Morante Martínez, P., & Dankloff Mora, C. (1993). Definición densitométrica de la morfología estructural del huesos del esqueleto humano, *Jano* XLV:637-640.

Gómez-Oliveros, L. (1962). *Lecciones de Anatomía Humana. Osteología. Tercera parte. Miembros.* Madrid. Marban.

Goto, A., Murase, T., Hashimoto, J., Oka, K., Yoshikawa, H. & Sugamoto, K. (2009). Morphologic análisis of the medulary canal in rheumatoid elbows, *Journal of Shoulder and Elbow Surgery*.18(1):33-37.

Griffith, JF., Genant, HK. (2008). Bone mass and architecture determination: state of the art, *Best practice & Research Clinical Endocrinology & Metabolism*.22(5):737-764.

Hepp, P., Josten, C. (2007). Biology and Biomechanics in Osteosynthesis of Proximal Humerus Fractures, *European Journal of Trauma and Emergency Surgery* 33(4):337-344.

Hvid, I., Jensen, NC., Bünger, C., Solund, K., Djurhuus, JC. (1985). Bone mineral assay: its relation to the mechanical strength of cancellous bone, *Engineering in Medicine* 14:79-83.

Kalkwarf, HJ., Laor, T & Bean JA. (2011). Fracture risk in children with forearm injury is associated with volumetric bone density and cortical area (by peripheral QCT) and areal bone density (by DXA), *Osteoporosis International* 22:607-616.

Kawashima, T. & Uhthoff HK. (1991). Pattern of bone loss of the proximal femur: a radiologic, densitometric, and histomorphometric study, *Journal of Orthopaedic Research* 9(5):630-640.

Kim, JM., Mudgal, CS., Konopka, JF & Júpiter JB. (2011). Complications of total elbow arthroplasty, *Journal of American Academy of Orthopaedic Surgeons.* 19(6):328-339.

McCarthy, CK., Steinberg, GG., Agren, M., Leahey, D., Wyman, E., & Baran DT (1991). Quantifying bone loss from the proximal femur after total hip arthroplasty, *Journal of Bone and Joint Surgery* 73(5):774-778.

Miralles Marrero, R. (1998). *Biomecánica Clínica del Aparato Locomotor.* Barcelona: Masson.

Pauwels, F. (1980) *Biomechanics of the Locomotor Apparatus. Contribution on the functional of the Locomotor Apparatus.* Nueva York: Srpinger.

Rettig, AC. (1983). Stress fracture of the ulna in an adolescent tournament tennis player. *American Journal of Sports Medicine* 11:103-106.

Sanchez-Sotelo, J. (2011). Total elbow arthroplasty, *The Open Orthopaedics Journal* 16(5):115-123.

Schoenau, E., Land, C., Stabrey, A., Remer, T. & Kroke, A. (2004). The bone mass concept: problems in short stature, *European Journal of Endocrinology* 151:S87-S91.

Testut, L. & Latarjet, A. (1949). *Tratado de Anatomía Humana. Volume 1* Barcelona: Salvat.

Tsujio, M., Mizorogi, T., Kitamura, I., Maeda, Y., Nishijima, K., Kuwahara, S., Ohno, T., Niida, S., Nagoya, M., Saito, R. & Tanaka, S. (2009). Bone mineral analisis through dual energy X-ray absorptiometry in laboratory animals, *Journal of Veterinary Medical Science* 71(11):1493-1497.

Viladot Voegeli, A. (2001) *Lecciones Básicas de Biomecánica del Aparato Locomotor.* Barcelona: Springer.

Wahner, HW., Eastell, R. & Riggs, BL. (1985). Bone mineral density of the radius: Where do we stand?, *The Journal of Nuclear Medicine* 26(11):1339-1341.

Weber, MF., Barbosa, DM., Belentani, C., Ramos, PM., Trudell, D. & Resnick, D. (2009). Coronoid process of the ulna: paleopathologic and anatomic study with imaging correlation. Emphasis on the anteromedial "facet", *Skeletal Radiology* 38(1):61-67.

8

Ex Vivo and *In Vivo* Assessment of Vertebral Strength and Vertebral Fracture Risk Assessed by Dual Energy X-Ray Absorptiometry

Kazuhiro Imai[1,2,3]
[1]*Department of Orthopaedic Surgery, Mishuku Hospital, Tokyo,*
[2]*Department of Orthopaedic Surgery, School of Medicine, Tokyo University,*
[3]*Department of Orthopaedic Surgery, Tokyo Metropolitan Geriatric Medical Center, Japan*

1. Introduction

Osteoporosis is defined as a skeletal disorder characterized by loss of bone mass, decreased bone strength and resulting in increased risk of bone fracture. The disease is progressive with age, especially in postmenopausal women [1]. Osteoporotic hip fractures and vertebral fractures have become a major social problem because the elderly population continues to increase. Hip fractures account for about 10% of all osteoporosis-related fractures [2]. Hip fractures are particularly devastating and have a particularly negative impact on morbidity. Survivors often suffer severe and prolonged physical and social limitations, and fail to recover normal activity [3]. Vertebral fractures affect approximately 25% of postmenopausal women [4]. Vertebral fractures can be associated with chronic disabling pain and incur loss of normal activity.

In addition to this increased awareness of osteoporosis as a significant health problem, there has been the emergence of several novel drugs that appear to be effective at reducing the risk of fracture, such as bisphosphonates. Consequently, clinicians and researchers are emphasizing the importance of early detection of osteoporosis, aggressive fracture prevention, and monitoring of patients who have high risk of fractures. Fracture risk associated with osteoporosis consisted of bone strength reduction and tendency to fall, therefore it is essential to measure bone strength to assess the risk of fracture. Bone strength reflects the integration of bone density and bone quality, which are influenced by bone architecture, bone turnover, accumulation of damage, and mineralization [5].

Traditionally, measurement of areal bone mineral density (aBMD) by dual energy X-ray absorptiometry (DXA) has served as the means by which to best diagnose osteoporosis and evaluate fracture risk [6]. In 1994, the World Health Organization (WHO) published a set of diagnostic criteria to define osteoporosis in postmenopausal Caucasian women, using aBMD values measured by DXA [7]. Measurement of aBMD by DXA has been the standard method for diagnosing osteoporosis, in addition to assessing fracture risk and therapeutic effects. However, a variety of problems exist with DXA, which include its relatively high cost, the absence of DXA in many communities, especially in less-developed countries.

Therefore, aBMD by DXA is not a suitable screening method for fracture risk in terms of accessibleness and cost. In addition, the correlations between bone strength and aBMD by DXA are reported to be 0.51-0.80 [8-11], which indicates aBMD only accounts for 50 to 80% of bone strength. And the application of aBMD measurements in isolation cannot identify individuals who eventually experience bone fracture because of the low sensitivity of the test [12].

Recently, quantitative ultrasound (QUS) is emerging as a relatively low-cost and readily accessible alternative means to identify osteoporosis, evaluate fracture risk, and initiate osteoporosis treatment. More recently, finite element (FE) method based on data from computed tomography (CT) has been used to assess bone strength, fracture risk, and therapeutic effects on osteoporosis.

2. Dual energy X-ray absorptiometry (DXA)

In the 1960s, a new method of measuring aBMD, called single-photon absorptiometry (SPA), was developed. In this method, a single-energy photon beam is passed through bone and soft tissue to a detector. The amount of mineral in the path is then quantified. This method most commonly uses a gamma-ray source coupled with a scintillation detector, which together scan across the area of interest [13]. The amount of the bone mineral in the tissue traversed by a well collimated gamma-ray beam is derived from its attenuation through bone plus soft tissue relative to that through soft tissue alone. The overall thickness of the soft tissue is standardized, usually by immersing the limb in water or cuffing with a fluid-filled bag. The value obtained is proportional to the bone mineral content of the segment scanned. The value may be divided by the bone width (yielding a result in g/cm) or by an estimate of the cross-sectional area to give a value for bone mineral density in g/cm^2. The technique has been applied to the femur, humerus, metacarpal, os calcis, hand and foot, but the most commonly used site is the forearm. The most frequently used source is ^{125}I (27keV), but has the major drawback of a relatively short half-life (60 days).

Accuracy may be compromised by a non-uniform thickness of fat, which has attenuation characteristics different from those of water or lean soft tissue. In some equipment, the program assumes the fat to be a uniform shell around the bone and makes a correction, but the correction requires a number of assumptions that influence the accuracy of the method. The heterogeneity of surrounding tissues is nevertheless considerably less than that of tissue surrounding axial sites such as the spine. Although true *in vivo* estimates of accuracy have not been made, errors in cadaveric studies of excised bone have sufficiently low to make the technique attractive for screening [14].

The radiation dose of SPA is very low and applied to a small volume of tissue, giving an effective dose equivalent of < 1μSv. Typical scanning times are 10-15 minutes. Single-energy X-ray absorptiometry (SXA) is a newly developed technique suitable for scanning appendicular sites. It avoids the need for isotopes and is likely to replace SPA.

The proximal femur and the vertebral bodies, with their associated processes, are very irregular bones that are difficult to delineate. Furthermore, they are surrounded by a widely varying amount of fat and muscle mass. The ratio of bone mass to soft tissue is thus lower in the spine or hip than in the forearm, and standardization of soft tissue by immersion in water is not feasible for these sites. These and other factors limit the use of SPA or SXA to the appendicular skeleton. The development of dual-photon absorptiometry (DPA) and, more recently, dual-energy X-ray absorptiometry (DXA) have resolved at least some of these problems. The different thickness of soft tissue can be accommodated by simultaneous measurement of the transmission of gamma-rays of two different energies, which makes the techniques applicable to any part of the body, but particularly the lumbar spine and hip.

The theory underlying DPA and DXA requires that there are only two components present - bone and soft tissue of uniform composition. In practice, fat forms a further component with attenuation characteristics that differ from those of water, muscle and most organs. A uniform layer of fat is unimportant, but fat is distributed non-uniformly in the region of the lumbar spine and may cause errors of up to 10% in spinal bone mineral. Errors can also be introduced by fat within the vertebral bone marrow.

Total body bone mineral can be measured by DPA, but instrumental problems are greater because of the wide range of count rates and the non-uniform distribution of fat, which introduces errors. However, total body bone mineral measured by neutron activation analysis. As with SPA, the radiation dose for DPA is low, the effective dose equivalent for part-body examinations being only a few microsieverts (μSv).

Recently, sources of gamma radiation have been replaced by X-ray generators. The necessary pairs of effective energies can be obtained either by K-edge filtering, using cerium or samarium, or by rapidly switching the generator potential. The advantages of these approaches are a higher beam intensity and therefore faster scan, improved spatial resolution with easier identification of vertebrae, and better precision. The absence of source decay also eliminates problems associated with decreasing count rates over the lifetime of the source.

Like DPA, DXA determines bone mineral density from an anterior-posterior image. The sites most commonly measured are the lumbar spine, generally L2-L4, including the intervertebral discs. Other sites include the hip, forearm, whole body and skeletal segments. The error in reproducibility *in vitro* is 1-2%. DXA has been reported to have a high short-term and long-term precision *in vivo*, which is about twice that of DPA. This has led to its widespread use in studies of osteoporosis.

A recent development has been scanning of the lumbar spine in the lateral position, which has the advantage of eliminating the posterior arch and the spines of the vertebrae as well as aortic calcification from the measurement. Its limitations are the increased soft tissue mass and overlap of the projected image by the ribs and pelvis, so that only one or two vertebrae are measured. Lateral scanning provides a measurement of vertebral depth which, together with the antero-posterior area, can provide a volumetric measurement for calculating bone mineral mass per unit volume. Whether this volumetric density measure is a better predictor of fracture is unknown. The technique may be useful in assessment of bone density in children, allowing accurate assessment of vertebral size. The precision error of measurement of the vertebral body and mid-slice *in vivo* is of the order of 2% [15]. DXA has now largely replaced DPA for screening because of its greater precision, ease of use and freedom from several technical artifacts. The WHO defines osteoporosis as a value for aBMD by DXA 2.5 standard deviation (SD) or more below the mean for young Caucasian adult women (T-score diagnostic criteria of -2.5), based on data that this criterion identified 30% of all postmenopausal women as having osteoporosis, more than half of whom would have sustained a prior fracture [7].

3. Quantitative computed tomography (QCT)

In quantitative computed tomography (QCT), a thin transverse slice through the body is imaged. Under appropriate conditions, the image can be quantified to give a measure of volumetric bone mineral density (vBMD) (mg/cm^3), and cancellous bone can be measured independently of surrounding cortical bone and aortic calcification. Developments have been concentrated in two directions: the construction of special equipment using a radionuclide source for measurements of the forearm, and the adaptation of X-ray CT machines installed for general radiology to measure vBMD. The attraction of the technique is that cancellous bone can be examined separately from cortical bone. It also gives a true value for mineral density (mg/cm^3) unlike other techniques.

A dedicated forearm scanner was first described in the mid 1970s [16,17]. The photon source is ^{125}I and is mounted in a gantry with a sodium iodide scintillation detector. A linear scan is performed at each of 48 angular positions. Computer reconstruction generates an image in which a region of interest in the cancellous bone of the distal ulna is selected. Since 1980s, QCT has been used as a means for non-invasive quantitative determination of bone mineral of the spine [18,19].

A lateral plane projection scan is necessary for precise slice positioning through the centers of the vertebrae. Comparison between the CT Hounsfield numbers and a calibration standard scanned simultaneously allows bone density to be expressed in terms of the equivalent concentration of the material of the standard. Regions of interest within the vertebral bodies are selected: circular, elliptical, rectangular or other chosen areas are selected to include all the cancellous bone just inside the cortex. The relationship between the observed CT number and the true attenuation coefficient is subject to short- and long-term variation, so that it is necessary to scan the patient and a calibration standard simultaneously. Recently, simple standards with fewer components based on suspensions of calcium hydroxyapatite in plastic have been adopted. Comparison between the standard and the Hounsfield numbers of the trabecular region of the vertebral bodies allows bone density to be expressed in terms of the equivalent concentration of the material of the standard.

Investigators reported the prediction of vertebral body compressive strength using QCT. In 1985, McBroom et al. [20] showed a strong positive correlation between QCT and apparent density of the vertebral trabecular bone but could find only suggestive, not quite significant, correlations between QCT and the vertebral body compressive strength. Cann et al. [21] showed that QCT evaluation of vertebral trabecular bone mineral density is a useful tool for determining the patients with increased risk of vertebral fracture. The positive correlations between QCT and vertebral body compressive strength in cadaver studies are 0.72-0.74 [22,23].

The biggest source of error in X-ray CT systems is fat within the bone marrow: accuracy errors of up to 30%. The accuracy can be improved by carrying out scans at two different potentials (dual energy techniques); typically, 80 and 120 kVp are used. Kalender et al. [24] claim an accuracy error of 5% *in vitro*, but errors *in vivo* are likely to be larger. The effective radiation doses equivalent for QCT are 0.3 mSv for single energy techniques and 1 mSv for dual energy techniques, respectively [25].

4. Quantitative ultrasound (QUS) bone assessment method

QUS bone assessment method has been recently introduced as an alternative for peripheral bone mass assessment, reflecting bone strength, bone density, and bone elasticity or fragility, and may be superior to aBMD by DXA [26]. The advantages of this method over X-ray-based techniques, which include low cost, portability, and no radiation exposure, have encouraged the use of this method for defining a stage of development of osteoporosis and evaluating bone fracture risk.

There are several reports for assessing bone conditions *in vivo* using QUS method and apparatus. QUS devices can be classified mostly into 3 groups, related to the type of ultrasound transmission. Trabecular sound transmission is best for measuring the heel [27]. Cortical transverse transmission currently only is used in phalanx contact devices [28]. And cortical axial transmission presently is being investigated for use in phalanges, the radius, and the tibia [28]. Heel devices currently appear to have the most clinical applications, where QUS are being used and evaluated for the prediction of fracture risk, the diagnosis of osteoporosis, the initiation of osteoporosis treatment, the monitoring of osteoporosis treatment, and osteoporosis case finding. For these purposes, the recommended parameter of interest in clinical routine is a composite score, e.g., heel stiffness index or Quantitative Ultrasound Index (QUI) combining the results of broad-band ultrasound attenuation (BUA) and speed of sound (SOS), as measured in meters per second.

At the present time, there is good evidence that QUS can discriminate those with osteoporotic fractures from age-matched controls without osteoporotic fracture [29,30]. The power of heel QUS to predict fracture observed in cross-sectional studies has been confirmed prospectively in some populations as defined by sex, age, and ethnic background. This is particularly true of heel QUS and for hip and spinal fractures. However, because of methodological issues, it is difficult to compare studies. Nonetheless, it is possible to make the following generations. Using QUS of the heel, the increase in relative risk for each standard deviation decrease in stiffness index (SI) is approximately 2.0 for the hip and spine and roughly 1.5 for all fractures combined [31-41].

The evidence from studies is good that the heel QUS SI using QUS devices is predictive of hip fracture risk in Caucasian and Asian women over age 55 and of any fracture risk in Asian women over age 55. Cortical axial transmission devices have no prospectively proven clinical utility, although clinical use in adults of phalanx QUS devices using cortical transverse transmission is also limited. These results for heel QUS are roughly the same as for DXA by BMD in terms of hip and spine fracture risk per SD decrease [12,42]. Discordant results between heel QUS and DXA, which are not infrequent, are not necessarily an indication of methodological error but rather due to the independence between the 2 techniques.

Diagnosing osteoporosis using QUS is less supported by evidence and more complicated and problematic than assessing fracture risk. To start with, the T-score diagnostic criteria of -2.5, classically used for DXA aBMD, cannot be applied to QUS without discrepancies in the numbers of women diagnosed with osteoporosis because of tremendous variations in QUS measurements by skeletal site, because different QUS devices yield different results, and because of the relatively poor correlation between heel QUS and hip/spine DXA measurements. If the prevalence of osteoporosis is defined as -2.5 SD from the mean threshold for QUS, even within the same sample population, different QUS instruments and different skeletal sites generate prevalence estimates that vary as much as 10-fold, such as prevalence estimates among Caucasian women over age 65 ranging from 4 to 50% [43-46]. To overcome this dilemma, there is a need for predefined, device-specific diagnostic thresholds. One recommended system suggests calibrating QUS measurements with DXA results, the latter used as the "gold standard," so that an upper QUS threshold is set to identify osteoporosis with 90% sensitivity and a lower threshold is set to identify osteoporosis with 90% specificity [47]. Using such a system, one could identify osteoporosis with high probability in patients whose results fall below the lower threshold for QUS, where specificity exceeds 90%; between the upper and lower thresholds, the diagnosis of osteoporosis would be considered quite equivocal, so that another means of measurement, like DXA aBMD, would be highly recommended; and above the upper threshold for QUS, where the sensitivity of a value below the threshold is 90%, osteoporosis would be deemed unlikely.

Except in the case of a low-energy fractures of the hip or spine, when the fracture alone is adequate to require treatment, all currently published recommendations for the initiation of treatment for osteoporosis are based on DXA aBMD values; in no instance, to date, are the results of QUS the definitive parameter. Despite this, several studies have demonstrated high levels of correlation between heel trabecular sound transmission and aBMD at matched skeletal sites [48-50]. Moreover, both SOS and BUA, standard QUS measurements, are dependent on overall bone strength which, in turn, is related to bone density, architecture and turnover, and the extent of bone mineralization [48,50,51-56]. These factors likely work together to maintain the overall quality and strength of bone and to prevent fractures and other bone failure. QUS parameters of heel trabecular transverse transmission are highly correlated with bone strength [57-62]. Consequently, it is conceivable that QUS guidelines for treatment initiation could be created, especially if combined with the use of clinical risk factors [63]. But no randomized clinical trials have been published examining whether individuals identified as high risk for fracture by QUS respond to treatment.

5. Finite element (FE) method based on data from computed tomography

The finite element (FE) method, an advanced computer technique of structural stress analysis developed in engineering mechanics, was first introduced to orthopaedic biomechanics in 1972 to evaluate stressed in human bones [64]. Since then, this method has been used to study the mechanics of human bones [65]. In the early 1990s, the FE method of analyzing a bone for fracture risk using 3-dimensional CT data was developed.

The object of this method is to measure non-invasively the strength of an individual bone in an individual patient. This measurement can then be used to determine whether or not the bone will fracture under specified loading conditions such as those normally seen in daily living. It can also be used to estimate fracture risks under abnormal loading conditions such as occur in falling, jumping or during athletic events or heavy training regimens. This method uses the distribution of physical properties of bone measured non-invasively in an individual and mathematical analysis of that distribution to predict the risk that a bone may fracture under applied loads. The use of such methods relates to the clinical disease of osteoporosis, or in general metabolic bone diseases. In a primary application, 3-dimensional CT data acquired using a conventional CT scanner are used to determine the distribution of bone mineral density, this distribution is used to define bone material properties, and the FE method of analysis is used to determine structural properties of the whole or a part of the bone. This information is then used to predict risk of fracture under specified loading conditions. Specifically, the distribution of bone material properties determined non-invasively is used as input to a FE analysis of structural strength, and other parameters such as loading conditions and boundary conditions are also included in the model as needed. Using mathematical methods contained in commercially-available or specially written computer programs, the model of a bone can be incrementally loaded until failure, and the yield strength determined.

A FE method based on data from CT has been applied to predict proximal femoral fracture [66-70]. CT-based FE method appears more predictive of femoral strength than QCT or DXA alone [66] and can predict proximal femoral fracture location [68]. Nonlinear FE method demonstrated improved predictions of femoral strength [69]. For the spine, CT-based nonlinear FE method was clinically applied to assess vertebral strength [71] and cadaver studies have been performed to evaluate the accuracy of CT-based FE method [72-77]. The cadaver studies have verified CT-based FE method predicts failure loads and fracture patterns for 10-mm-thick vertebral sections [72] and can predict *ex vivo* vertebral compressive strength better than aBMD [73,74] and QCT alone [75]. CT-based nonlinear FE method can accurately predict vertebral strength, fracture sites and distribution of minimum principal strain *ex vivo* [77]. Based on verification by the cadaver studies, FE method has been applied clinically to the assessment of chronic glucocorticoid treatment at the hip [78], as well as teriparatide and alendronate treatment for osteoporosis at the lumbar spine [79], proving useful for assessing medication effects on bone strength.

A study assessing vertebral fracture risk and medication effects on osteoporosis *in vivo* with CT-based nonlinear FE method showed that analyzed vertebral compressive strength had stronger discriminatory power for vertebral fracture than aBMD and vBMD, and detected alendronate effects at 3 months earlier than aBMD and vBMD [80]. The CV (coefficient of variation) for the measurement of vertebral compressive strength was 0.96% *ex vivo*. The effective radiation dose for assessing vertebral compressive strength is 3 mSv.

CT-based FE method predicts compressive bone strength accurately and is useful for assessing the risk of fracture and therapeutic effects on osteoporosis, and provides unique theories from a biomechanical perspective. This method also predicts bone strength under specified loading conditions such as those normally seen in activities of daily living [81,82].

6. Assessment of vertebral strength *ex vivo* by DXA

This study was conducted at Tokyo University in Tokyo, Japan. The study protocol was approved by the ethics committee.

Twelve thoracolumbar (T11, T12, and L1) vertebrae with no skeletal pathologies were collected within 24 hours of death from 4 males (31, 55, 67, and 83 years old). Causes of death for the four donors were myelodysplastic syndrome, pneumonia, adult T-cell leukemia, and bladder cancer, respectively. All of the specimens were obtained at Tokyo University Hospital with the approval of the ethics committee and with informed consent. They were stored at -70 C° after each step in the protocol. The vertebrae were disarticulated, and the discs were excised. Then the posterior elements of each vertebra were removed by cutting through the pedicles. The vertebrae were immersed in water and aBMD (g/cm^2) of the vertebrae were measured by DXA (DPX; Lunar, Madison, WI, USA) in the supine position.

To assess vertebral strength, a quasi-static uniaxial compression test of each vertebra was conducted. To restrain the specimens for load testing, both upper and lower surfaces of the vertebrae were embedded in dental resin (Ostron; GC Dental Products Co., Aichi, Japan) so that the two surfaces were exactly parallel. Then the embedded specimens were placed on a mechanical testing machine (TENSILON UTM-2.5T; Orientec, Tokyo, Japan) and were compressed at a cross-head displacement rate of 0.5 mm per minute. A compression plate with a ball joint was used to apply a uniform load onto the upper surface of the specimen. The applied load was measured by a load cell (T-CLB-5-F-SR; T. S. Engineering, Kanagawa, Japan). The load was recorded using MacLab/4 (AD Instruments, Castle Hill, NSW, Australia) at a sampling rate of 2 Hz. The measured vertebral strength was defined as the ultimate load achieved. Pearson's correlation analysis was used to evaluate correlations between the measured aBMD by DXA and the measured vertebral strength by mechanical testing.

The result from the *ex vivo* assessment, aBMD by DXA ranged from 0.287 to 0.705 g/cm^2, while the measured vertebral strength by mechanical testing ranged from 1.54 to 4.62 kN. There were significant linear correlations between aBMD and the measured vertebral strength ($r = 0.915$, $p < 0.0001$) (Fig. 1).

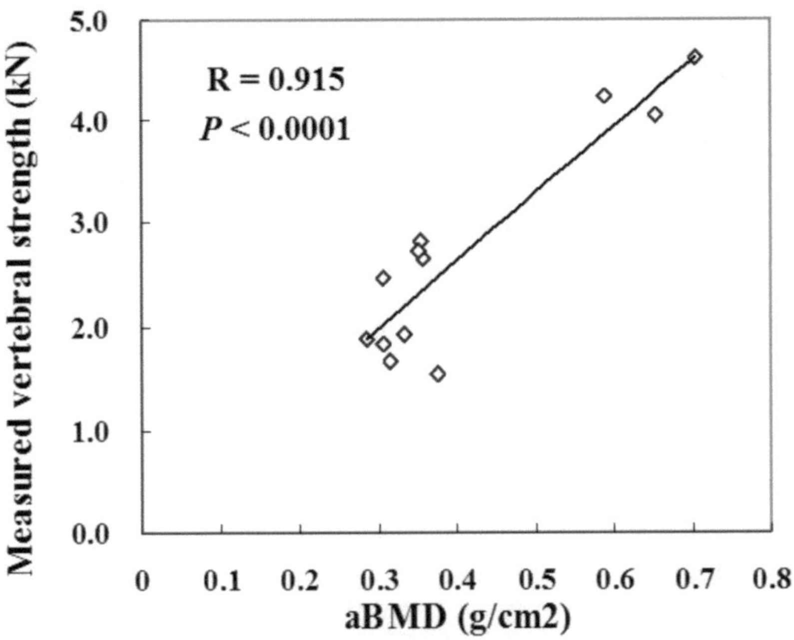

Fig. 1. The experimentally measured vertebral strength versus aBMD measured by DXA. They were significantly correlated.

7. Assessment of vertebral fracture risk *in vivo* by DXA

This study was conducted at Tokyo Metropolitan Geriatric Medical Center in Tokyo, Japan. The study protocol was approved by the ethics committee and each participant provided written informed consent in accordance with the Declaration of Helsinki.

The inclusion criteria included ambulatory postmenopausal Japanese women aged between 49 and 85 years old. Exclusion criteria included women with any disorders of bone and mineral metabolism other than postmenopausal osteoporosis, those who had any recent or current treatment with the potential to alter bone turnover or bone metabolism. Vertebral fracture was diagnosed based on lateral spine radiography. Radiographic vertebral fracture was defined if either the anterior or central height was ≥20% less than posterior height. A total of 123 eligible participants were enrolled in this cross-sectional study. For all participants, aBMD of the anteroposterior (AP) lumbar spine (L2-4) were measured by DXA (DPX; Lunar, Madison, WI, USA).

Logistic regression analysis was performed to estimate risk factors for vertebral fracture. L2-4 aBMD was assessed using sensitivity and specificity curves to determine the optimal cut-off point as the vertebral fracture threshold. For each statistical analysis, differences were considered significant at $p<0.05$. Statistical analysis was performed using StatView for Windows version 5.0 software (SAS Institute, Cary, NC, USA).

The 123 women enrolled in the *in vivo* clinical study had a mean age of 71.8 ±7.4 years, mean height of 149.4 ±5.6 cm, and mean weight of 50.2 ±7.4 kg. Measured L2-4 aBMD was 0.816 ±0.191 g/cm^2. Subjects were classified on the basis of prior vertebral fracture. Among the 123 women, 75 subjects did not have any vertebral fractures (nonfracture group) and 48 subjects already had vertebral fractures (fracture group). The average aBMD of the non-fracture group was 0.860 ± 0.166 g/cm^2, which was greater than that of the fracture group at 0.759 ± 0.207 g/cm^2 (Mann-Whitney *U* test, $p = 0.0255$).

Vertebral fractures were present in 39.0% of the total study population. Among the fracture group, vertebral fractures spontaneously developed in 29 women (spontaneous fracture group) and were caused by trauma in 19 women (traumatic fracture group). Among the 19 subjects in the traumatic fracture group, 18 women developed fracture following a fall from standing height, and 1 woman developed fracture following a fall down stairs. To exclude factors of trauma, 75 subjects in the nonfracture group and 29 subjects in the spontaneous fracture group were compared. aBMD (Mann-Whitney *U* test, $p=0.0033$) was significantly decreased in the spontaneous fracture group compared with the nonfracture group. Logistic regression analysis after adjustment for age and body weight revealed that aBMD reduction as risk factors associated with spontaneous vertebral fracture, the odds ratio per SD decrease was 1.83 with 1.13-3.26 of 95% confidence interval ($p=0.0238$). aBMD was also assessed by sensitivity and specificity curves. The nonfracture group and spontaneous fracture group (104 women in total) were assessed in a cross-sectional manner. The optimal point on the sensitivity and specificity curves used as the fracture threshold to predict spontaneous vertebral fractures for aBMD was 0.816 g/cm^2 with 69.0% sensitivity and 72.0% specificity (Fig. 2).

8. Discussion

Bone strength primarily reflects bone density and bone quality, which are influenced by bone architecture, turnover, accumulation of damage, and mineralization [5]. Previous

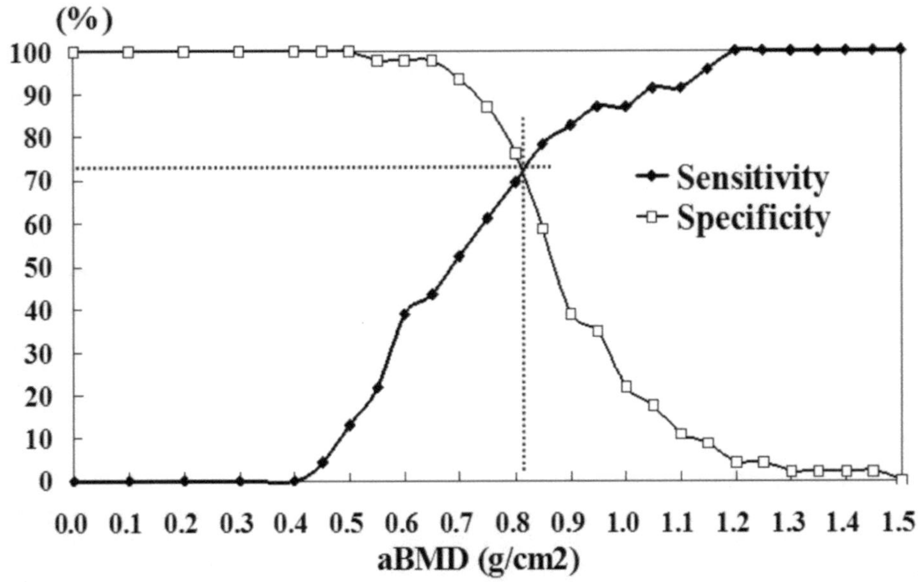

Fig. 2. Sensitivity and specificity curves to determine the optimal cut-off point of aBMD measured by DXA to predict spontaneous vertebral fracture.

studies showed that aBMD explained 50-80% of vertebral strength [8-11] based on data that the correlations between aBMD and the measured vertebral strength were 0.51 to 0.80. In this study, the correlations between the measured values of aBMD and the vertebral strength were 0.915 and better than the previous studies. This *ex vivo* study showed that aBMD measurements in isolation might assess vertebral strength well.

In the treatment of osteoporosis, the target is to assess fracture risk and prevent fractures. This *in vivo* study showed that aBMD had high discriminatory power for spontaneous vertebral fracture. The cut-off value of aBMD for predicting vertebral fractures without trauma was 0.816 g/cm^2, equivalent to -2.62 SD compared to young healthy Japanese women. Low trauma fractures such as a fall from a standing height are due to osteoporosis. The present assessment excluded the traumatic fracture group. Therefore, the threshold value was not for diagnosing osteoporosis, but for assessing spontaneous vertebral fracture risk.

This *ex vivo* and *in vivo* study showed that aBMD was a good parameter of vertebral strength and vertebral fracture risk. However, aBMD in isolation can only assess bone density and can not assess bone quality. Therefore, accuracy of assessing vertebral strength by aBMD is limited.

To improve accuracy of assessing vertebral strength and vertebral fracture risk, new method has been developed. CT-based nonlinear FE method can accurately predict vertebral strength, fracture sites and distribution of minimum principal strain *ex vivo* [77]. Based on verification by the cadaver studies, FE method has been applied clinically. A study assessing vertebral fracture risk and medication effects on osteoporosis *in vivo* with CT-based nonlinear FE method showed that analyzed vertebral compressive strength had stronger discriminatory power for vertebral fracture than aBMD and detected alendronate effects at 3 months earlier than aBMD [80].

This method assesses bone geometry and heterogeneous bone mass distribution as well as aBMD, but cannot detect microdamage and bone turnover. In clinical application, other parameters such as age and bone turnover markers should be included to assess the risk of fracture and therapeutic effects. Methods for assessing fracture risk and therapeutic effects on osteoporosis in the future might include other parameters as well as CT data.

Prediction by FE method with a smaller element size using the data from CT scans with a thinner slice thickness and a smaller pixel size is more accurate. On the other hand, thinner CT slices lead to more radiation exposure in the clinical situation. To decrease radiation exposure as much as possible during CT scanning, optimization of the element size of the FE method was performed by assessing the accuracy of the FE method simulation [83]. With the limited resolution of currently available CT scanners, the micro-architecture of the bone cannot be precisely assessed. Micro-CT and synchrotron micro-CT visualize bone microstructure. However, obtaining micro-CT scans of a whole vertebra *in vivo* would be impossible with the currently available scanners. Also, use of thinner CT slices to obtain images leads to more radiation exposure. With future developments, FE method based on micro-CT data with less radiation dose might be promising.

9. References

[1] Cummings SR, Kelsey JL, Nevitt MC, O'Dowd KJ. Epidemiology of osteoporosis and osteoporotic fractures. Epidemiol Rev. 1985;7:178-208.

[2] Eastell R, Reid DM, Compston J, *et al.* Secondary prevention of osteoporosis: when should a non-vertebral fracture be a trigger for action? Q J Med 2001;94:575-597.

[3] Wolinsky FD, Fitzgerald JF, Stump TE. The effect of hip fracture on mortality, hospitalization, and functional status: a prospective study. Am J Public Health 1997;87:398-403.

[4] Melton LJ 3rd. Epidemiology of spinal osteoporosis. Spine 1997;22(suppl):2-11.

[5] NIH Consensus Development Panel on Osteoporosis Prevention, Diagnosis, and Therapy. Osteoporosis prevention, diagnosis, and therapy. JAMA 2001;285:785-795.

[6] Kanis JA, Delmas P, Burckhardt P, Cooper C, Torgerson D. Guidelines for diagnosis and management of osteoporosis. The European Foundation for Osteoporosis and Bone Disease. Osteoporos Int. 1997;7:390-406.

[7] World Health Organization. Assessment of fracture risk and its application to screening for postmenopausal osteoporosis. Report of a WHO Study Group. World Health Organ Tech Rep Ser 1994;843:1-129.

[8] Edmondston SJ, Singer KP, Day RE, *et al.* In-vitro relationships between vertebral body density, size and compressive strength in the elderly thoracolumbar spine. Clin Biomecha 1994; 9: 180-186.

[9] Cheng XG, Nicholson PH, Boonen S, *et al.* Prediction of vertebral strength in vitro by spinal bone densitometry and calcaneal ultrasound. J Bone Miner Res 1997;12:1721-1728.

[10] Myers BS, Arbogast KB, Lobaugh B, Harper KD, Richardson WJ, Drezner MK. Improved assessment of lumbar vertebral body strength using supine lateral dual-energy x-ray absorptiometry. J Bone Miner Res 1994;9:687-693.

[11] Bjarnason K, Hassager C, Svendsen OL, Stang H, Christiansen C. Anteroposterior and lateral spinal DXA for the assessment of vertebral body strength: comparison with hip and forearm measurement. Osteoporosis Int 1996;6:37-42.
[12] Marshall D, Johnell O, Wedel H. Meta-analysis of how well measures of bone mineral density predict occurrence of osteoporotic fractures. BMJ 1996;312:1254-1259.
[13] Vogel JM. Bone mineral measurement: Skylab experiment M-078. Acta Astronaut 1975;2:129-139.
[14] Oyster N, Smith FW. A postmortem correlation of four techniques of assessment of osteoporosis with force of bone compression. Calcif Tissue Int 1988;43:77-82.
[15] Uebelhart D, Duboeuf F, Meunier PJ, Delmas PD. Lateral dual-photon absorptiometry: a new technique to measure the bone mineral density at the lumbar spine. J Bone Miner Res 1990;5:525-531.
[16] Rüegsegger P, Elsasser U, Anliker M, Gnehm H, Kind H, Prader A. Quantification of bone mineralization using computed tomography. Radiology 1976;121:93-97.
[17] Isherwood I, Rutherford RA, Pullan BR, Adams PH. Bone-mineral estimation by computer-assisted transverse axial tomography. Lancet 1976;2:712-715.
[18] Genant HK, Boyd D, Rosenfeld D, Abols Y, Cann CE. Computed tomography. Non-invasive measurements of bone mass and their clinical application. Florida, CRC Press 1981;121-149.
[19] Powell MR, Kolb FO, Genant HK, Cann CE, Stebler BG. Comparison of dual photon absorbtiometry and quantitative computer tomography of the lumbar spine in the same subjects. Clinical disorders of bone and mineral metabolism. Amsterdam, Excerpta Medica 1983;58-60.
[20] McBroom RJ, Hayes WC, Edwards WT, *et al.* Prediction of vertebral body compressive fracture using quantitative computed tomography. J Bone Joint Surg 1985;67-A:1206-1214.
[21] Cann CE, Genant HK, Kolb FO, Ettinger B. Quantitative computed tomography for prediction of vertebral fracture risk. Bone 1985;6:1-7.
[22] Mosekilde L, Bentzen SM, Ortoft G, Jorgensen J. The predictive value of quantitative computed tomography for vertebral body compressive strength and ash density. Bone 1989;10:465-470.
[23] Eriksson SA, Isberg BO, Lindgren JU. Prediction of vertebral strength by dual photon absorptiometry and quantitative computed tomography. Calcif Tissue Int 1989;44:243-250.
[24] Kalender WA, Klotz E, Suess C. Vertebral bone mineral analysis: an integrated approach with CT. Radiology 1987;164:419-423.
[25] Huda W, Morin RL. Patient doses in bone mineral densitometry. Br J Radiol 1996;69:422-425.
[26] Hans D, Arlot ME, Schott AM, Roux JP, Kotzki PO, Meunier PJ. Do ultrasound measurements on the os calcis reflect more the bone microarchitecture than the bone mass? A two-dimensional histomorphometric study. Bone 1995;16:295-300.
[27] Njeh CF, Hans D, Fuerst T, Gluer CC, Genant HK (ed.), Quantitative ultrasound: assessment of osteoporisis and bone status - Calcaneal quantitative ultrasound. London, Martin Dunitz. 1999;109-144.

[28] Njeh CF, Hans D, Fuerst T, Gluer CC, Genant HK (ed.), Quantitative ultrasound: assessment of osteoporisis and bone status - Non-heel quantitative ultrasound devices. London, Martin Dunitz. 1999;145-162.
[29] Durosier C, Hans D, Krieg MA, Schott AM. Prediction and discrimination of osteoporotic hip fracture in postmenopausal women. J Clin Densitom 2006;9:475-495.
[30] Krieg MA, Barkmann R, Gonnelli S, *et al.* Quantitative ultrasound in the management of osteoporosis: The 2007 ISCD official positions. J Clin Densitom Assess Skelet Health 2008;11:163-187.
[31] Porter RW, Miller CG, Grainger D, Palmer SB. Prediction of hip fracture in elderly women: A prospective study. BMJ 1990;301:638-641.
[32] Heaney RP, Avioli LV, Chesnut CH 3rd, Lappe J, Recker RR, Brandenburger GH. Ultrasound velocity, through bone predicts incident vertebral deformity. J Bone Miner Res 1995;10:341-345.
[33] Hans D, Dargent-Molina P, Schott AM, *et al.* Ultrasonographic heel measurements to predict hip fracture in elderly women: The EPIDOS prospective study. Lancet 1996;348:511-514.
[34] Bauer DC, Gluer CC, Cauley JA, *et al.* Broadband ultrasound attenuation predicts fractures strongly and independently of densitometry in older women. A prospective study. Study of Osteoporotic Fractures Research Group. Arch Intern Med 1997;157:629-634.
[35] Pluijm SM, Graafmans WC, Bouter LM, Lips P. Ultrasound measurements for the prediction of osteoporotic fractures in elderly people. Osteoporos Int 1999;9:550-556.
[36] Fujiwara S, Sone T, Yamazaki K, *et al.* Heel bone ultrasound predicts non-spine fracture in Japanese men and women. Osteoporos int 2005;16:2107-2112.
[37] Schott AM, Hans D, Duboeuf F, *et al.* Quantitative ultrasound parameters as well as bone mineral density are better predictors of trochanteric than cervical hip fractures in elderly women. Results from the EPIDOS study. Bone 2005;37:858-863.
[38] Gluer MG, Minne HW, Gluer CC, *et al.* Prospective identification of postmenopausal osteoporotic women at high vertebral fracture risk by radiography, bone densitometry, quantitative ultrasound, and laboratory findings: results from the PIOS study. J Clin Densitom 2005;8:386-395.
[39] Krieg MA, Cornuz J, Ruffieux C, *et al.* Prediction of hip fracture risk by quantitative ultrasound in more than 7000 Swiss women > or = 70 years of age: Comparison of three technologically different bone ultrasound devices in the SEMOF study. J Bone Miner Res 2006;21:1457-1463.
[40] Diez-Perez, Gonzalez-Macias, Marin F, *et al.* Prediction of absolute risk of non-spinal fractures using clinical risk factors and heel quantitative ultrasound. Osteoporos Int 2007;18:629-639.
[41] Bauer DC, Ewing S, Cauley J, Ensrud K, Cummings S, Orwoll E. Quantitative ultrasound predicts hip and non-spine fracture in men: The MrOS study. Osteoporos Int 2007;18:771-777.
[42] Durosier C, Hans D, Krieg MA, Schott AM. Prediction and discrimination of osteoporotic hip fracture in postmenopausal women. J Clin Densitom 2006;9:475-495.

[43] Frost ML, Blake GM, Fogelman I. Can the WHO criteria for diagnosing osteoporosis be applied to calcaneal quantitative ultrasound? Osteoporosis Int 2000;11:321-330.

[44] Faulkner KG, von Stetten E, Miller P. Discordance in patient classification using T-scores. J Clin Densitom 1999;2:343-350.

[45] Damilakis J, Perisinakis K, Gourtsoyiannis N. Imaging ultrasonometry of the calcaneus: Optimum T-score thresholds for the identification of osteoporotic subjects. Calcif Tissue Int 2001;68:219-224.

[46] Knapp KM, Blake GM, Spector TD, Fogelman I. Can the WHO definition of osteoporosis be applied to multisite axial transmission quantitative ultrasound? Osteoporosis Int 2004;15:367-374.

[47] Clowes JA, Peel NF, Eastell R. Device-specific thresholds to diagnose osteoporosis at the proximal femur: An approach to interpreting peripheral bone measurements in clinical practice. Osteoporosis Int 2006;17:1293-1302.

[48] Siffert RS, Kaufman JJ. Ultrasonic bone assessment: The time has come. Bone 2007;40:5-8.

[49] Roux C, Fournier B, Laugier P, *et al.* Broadband ultrasound attenuation imaging: A new imaging method in osteoporosis. J Bone Miner Res 1996;11:1112-1118.

[50] Hans D, Arlot ME, Schott AM, Roux JP, Kotzki PO, Meunier PJ. Do ultrasound measurements on the os calcis reflect more the bone microarchitecture than the bone mass?: A two-dimensional histomorphometric study. Bone 1995;16:295-300.

[51] Seeman E, Delmas PD. Bone quality - the material and structural basis of bone strength and fragility. N Engl J Med 2006;354:2250-2261.

[52] Ammann P, Rizzoli R. Bone strength and its determinants. Osteoporosis Int 2003;14:S13-S18.

[53] Hans D, Wu C, Njeh CF, *et al.* Ultrasound velocity of trabecular cubes reflects mainly bone density and elasticity. Calcif Tissue Int 1999;64:18-23.

[54] Gluer CC. Quantitative ultrasound - it is time to focus research efforts. Bone 2007;40:9-13.

[55] Gluer CC, Wu CY, Genant HK. Broadband ultrasound attenuation signals depend on trabecular orientation: An *in vitro* study. Osteoporosis Int 1993;3:185-191.

[56] Gluer CC, Wu CY, Jergas M, Goldstein SA, Genant HK. Three quantitative ultrasound parameters reflect bone structure. Calcif Tissue Int 1994;55:46-52.

[57] Bouxsein ML, Coan BS, Lee SC. Prediction of the strength of the elderly proximal femur by bone mineral density and quantitative ultrasound measurements of the heel and tibia. Bone 1999;25:49-54.

[58] Bouxsein ML, Radloff SE. Quantitative ultrasound of the calcaneus reflects the mechanical properties of calcaneal trabecular bone. J Bone Miner Res 1997;12:839-846.

[59] Lochmuller EM, Burklein D, Kuhn V, *et al.* Mechanical strength of the thoracolumbar spine in the elderly: Prediction from in situ dual-energy X-ray absorptiometry, quantitative computed tomography, upper and lower limb peripheral quantitative computed tomography, and quantitative ultrasound. Bone 2002;31:77-84.

[60] Hakulinen MA, Toyras J, Saarakkala S, Hirvonen J, Kroger H, Jurvelin JS. Ability of ultrasound backscattering to predict mechanical properties of bovine trabecular bone. Ultrasound Med Biol 2004;30:919-927.

[61] Han S, Medige J, Faran K, Feng Z, Ziv I. The ability of quantitative ultrasound to predict the mechanical properties of trabecular bone under different strain rates. Med Eng Phys 1997;19:742-747.

[62] Njeh CF, Kuo CW, Langton CM, Atrah HI, Boivin CM. Prediction of human femoral bone strength using ultrasound velocity and BMD. An *in vitro* study. Osteoporosis Int 1997;7:471-477.

[63] Durosier C, Hans D, Krieg MA, *et al.* Combining clinical factors and quantitative ultrasound improves the detection of women both at low and high risk for hip fracture. Osteoporosis Int 2007;18:1651-1659.

[64] Brekelmans WA, Poort HW, Slooff TJ. A new method to analyse the mechanical behaviour of skeletal parts. Acta Orthop Scand 1972;43:301-317.

[65] Huiskes R, Chao EY. A survey of finite element analysis in orthopedic biomechanics: the first decade. J Biomech 1983;16:385-409.

[66] Cody DD, Gross GJ, Hou FJ, *et al.* Femoral strength is better predicted by finite element models than QCT and DXA. J Biomech 1999;32:1013-1020.

[67] Keyak JH, Rossi SA, Jones KA, *et al.* Prediction of femoral fracture load using automated finite element modeling. J Biomech 1998;31:125-133.

[68] Keyak JH, Rossi SA, Jones KA, *et al.* Prediction of fracture location in the proximal femur using finite element models. Med Eng Phys 2001;23:657-664.

[69] Keyak JH. Improved prediction of proximal femoral fracture load using nonlinear finite element models. Med Eng Phys 2001;23:165-173.

[70] Bessho M, Ohnishi I, Matsuyama J, *et al.* Prediction of strength and strain of the proximal femur by a CT-based finite element method. J Biomech 2007;40:1745-1753.

[71] Faulkner KG, Cann CE, Hasegawa BH. Effect of bone distribution on vertebral strength: assessment with patient-specific nonlinear finite element analysis. Radiology 1991;179:669-674.

[72] Silva MJ, Keaveny TM, Hayes WC. Computed tomography-based finite element analysis predicts failure loads and fracture patterns for vertebral sections. J Orthop Res 1998;16:300-308.

[73] Martin H, Werner J, Andresen R, *et al.* Noninvasive assessment of stiffness and failure load of human vertebrae from CT-data. Biomed Tech 1998;43:82-88.

[74] Buckley JM, Loo K, Motherway J. Comparison of quantitative computed tomography-based measures in predicting vertebral strength. Bone 2007;40:767-774.

[75] Crawford RP, Cann CE, Keaveny TM. Finite element models predict in vitro vertebral body compressive strength better than quantitative computed tomography. Bone 2003;33:744-750.

[76] Liebschner MA, Kopperdahl DL, Rosenberg D, *et al.* Finite element modeling of the human thoracolumbar spine. Spine 2003;28:559-565.

[77] Imai K, Ohnishi I, Bessho M, *et al.* Nonlinear finite element model predicts vertebral bone strength and fracture site. Spine 2006;31:1789-1794.

[78] Lian KC, Lang TF, Keyak JH, *et al.* Differences in hip quantitative computed tomography (QCT) measurements of bone mineral density and bone strength between glucocorticoid-treated and glucocorticoid-naive postmenopausal women. Osteoporos Int 2005;16:642-650.

[79] Keaveny TM, Donley DW, Hoffmann PF, *et al.* Effects of teriparatide and alendronate on vertebral strength as assessed by finite element modeling of QCT scans in women with osteoporosis. J Bone Miner Res 2007;22:149-157.

[80] Imai K, Ohnishi I, Matsumoto T, Yamamoto S, Nakamura K. Assessment of vertebral fracture risk and therapeutic effects of alendronate in postmenopausal women using a quantitative computed tomography-based nonlinear finite element method. Osteoporosis Int 2009;20:801-810.

[81] Matsumoto T, Ohnishi I, Bessho M, Imai K, Ohashi S, Nakamura K. Prediction of vertebral strength under loading conditions occurring in activities of daily living using a computed tomography-based nonlinear finite element method. Spine 2009;34:1464-1469.

[82] Bessho M, Ohnishi I, Matsumoto T, *et al.* Prediction of proximal femur strength using a CT-based nonlinear finite element method: differences in predicted fracture load and site with changing load and boundary conditions. Bone 2009;45:226-231.

[83] Imai K, Ohnishi I, Yamamoto S, Nakamura K. *In vivo* assessment of lumbar vertebral strength in elderly women using computed tomography-based nonlinear finite element model. Spine 2008;33:27-32.

9

Dietary Protein and Bone Health

Anne Blais, Emilien Rouy and Daniel Tomé
UMR-914 INRA-AgroParisTech, Nutrition Physiology and Ingestive Behavior, Paris, France

1. Introduction

Dietary proteins represent 10 to 20% of energy consumption. The recommended daily minimum intake of protein and amino acids in adults is 0.8 g per kg of body weight. However, no upper limit has been identified. In industrialized countries, the main sources of protein are milk, eggs and meat. The nutritional value of protein is influenced by several factors, especially the amino acid (AA) composition, protein digestibility, protein digestion kinetics and the ability to transfer AA for protein synthesis. Diets based on either animal or vegetable products supply proteins of differing quality in differing quantities. Plant proteins are often deficient or low in some specific indispensable AAs. Soy protein is reported as a "complete" protein but its overall indispensable AA content is relatively low (~85% lower than milk) (Wilson & Wilson, 2006).

Epidemiological data support a positive association between protein intake and bone health. Protein is the precursor of AAs used for bone matrix protein synthesis. Moreover, studies evaluating the relationship between dietary protein and bone turnover support the hypothesis that high protein intake may decrease bone resorption. IGF-1 is a key mediator of bone growth (Geusens & Boonen, 2002) and dietary protein is an important regulator of circulating IGF-1 levels (Bonjour *et al.*, 2001). However, protein is also known to be calciuric, though the origin of the increased calcium excretion is debated. According to the acid ash hypothesis, the protein-induced acid load would have a deleterious effect on bone (Barzel & Massey, 1998). Finally, some proteins, due to their amino acid content, have specific effects on bone metabolism by acting directly on bone cells or through indirect pathways.

Even if the effect of nutrition on bone is not as dramatic as that of pharmaceuticals, it can be of great help when considering bone loss. Indeed nutrition is a lower-cost, longer-term, higher-compliance and wider-spread approach than pharmaceutical treatment. The nutritional intervention can be done alone preventively or in combination with a therapy in more severe cases. Some nutritional components such as calcium and vitamin D are recognized to have a positive effect on bone. However, the effect of protein on bone health is much more debated.

This chapter reviews the literature on the subject, giving an overview of the data available and comparing the proposed mechanisms of action. Attention is drawn to protein quality and to the specific effect of some soy, collagen and milk peptides on bone metabolism.

2. Action of protein on bone

The mechanism underlying the debate on the effect of protein on bone is the hormonal anabolic effect. It is based on the increase of bone anabolic hormone IGF-1 with the consumption of protein.

2.1 Bone protein metabolism and turnover

Type I collagen is the major structural protein distributed throughout the whole body accounting for 25% of total body protein and for 80% of total conjunctive tissue in humans. The different factors involved in bone strength include not only mineral density, crystal characteristics, micro architecture, geometry and morphology (size and shape), but also protein matrix and collagen fiber quality. Cortical bone strength, whose main role is to protect bone integrity, is influenced not only by porosity, presence of micro damage and mineral composition, but also by the orientation of collagen fibers, extent and nature of collagen cross-linking and number and composition of cement lines (Burr, 2002; Currey, 2001; Seeman & Delmas, 2006; Turner, 2006). Collagen is an important component of bone, being the main extra cellular matrix protein for calcification and playing a role in osteoblast differentiation (Takeuchi *et al.*, 1996, 1997).

Markers of bone resorption, which measure the release of peptide resulting of the degradation of mature modified type 1 collagen into the serum and urine, are commonly used to evaluate the relationship between dietary protein and bone turnover. However, to better understand the effect of feeding on bone collagen turnover, a better knowledge of the physiology of bone collagen synthesis is needed (Babraj Smith 2005).

2.2 Hormonal anabolic effect

Protein has an anabolic effect on bone metabolism by upregulating Insulin-like Growth Factor 1 (IGF-1). IGF-1 is a peptide hormone mainly produced by the liver under the action of the Growth Hormone. A small percentage of IGF-1 is also produced locally by different cell types throughout the body, including osteoblasts (Ohlsson *et al.*, 2009). There is good evidence of the anabolic effect of IGF-1 on bone and muscle, especially when considering age-related disorders (Perrini *et al.*, 2010). Studies measuring IGF-1 levels under different protein intakes consistently report that a high protein intake increases IGF-1. This fact has been shown over a six-month period in young exercising subjects (Ballard *et al.*, 2005) and evidence also exists in older populations of both sexes (Arjmandi *et al.*, 2005; Dawson-Hughes *et al.*, 2004; Hunt *et al.*, 2009).

There is some evidence that this hormonal response is based on the quality of the protein ingested. Dawson-Hughes and colleagues showed that a fivefold increase of aromatic AA intake (phenylalanine and histidine) for 24 days induced an increase of IGF-1 level. On the other hand, a fivefold increase of branched chain AA (leucine and isoleuine) induced no effect on IGF-1, indicating that the protein intake effect on IGF-1 is probably AA-dependent (Dawson-Hughes *et al.*, 2007). Moreover, two studies comparing milk and soy protein reported that soy induces a greater increase of IGF-1 (Arjmandi *et al.*, 2003; Khalil *et al.*, 2002). However, it is important to note that the soy protein contained isoflavone in both studies, thus the effect on IGF-1 could be attributed to this molecule rather than to the AA content.

The effect of protein intake on IGF-1 level could involve Calcium-Sensing Receptor (CaSR) which was also reported to be implicated in the calciuric effect of protein (Conigrave *et al.*, 2008). *In vitro* investigations showed that CaSR is expressed in hepatocytes (Canaff *et al.*, 2001). The activation of CaSR in the liver by AA could explain the increased IGF-1 level due to protein consumption. Moreover, osteoblasts also express CaSR and produce IGF-1 under its regulation. CaSR also upregulates numerous bone forming mechanisms and inhibits bone resorption (Marie, 2010). Aromatic AA supplementation induces an increase in IGF-1 while branched chain AAs have no effect (Dawson-Hughes *et al.*, 2007). This is consistent with the findings of Conigrave *et al.*, that aromatic AAs are the most potent activators of CaSR, while branched chain AAs are the less potent ones (Conigrave *et al.*, 2000).

There is no doubt that protein induces an increase of IGF-1 level. By doing so and according to what is known of IGF-1, protein is likely to have an anabolic effect on bone. The proposed mechanism would be that a high protein intake (especially one rich in aromatic AAs) would activate CaSR in hepatocytes and osteoblasts and stimulate IGF-1 production, which would in turn exert an anabolic effect on bone.

2.3 Bone turnover markers

Bone turnover markers are measured in blood or urine; they give information on bone formation or on bone resorption. Both types of markers are needed in a study in order to assess bone turnover.

The recent meta-analysis of Darling *et al.* concludes that there is no clear evidence of an effect of protein intake on bone markers (Darling *et al.*, 2009). Some studies reported an increase in bone resorption while bone formation remained stable (Kerstetter *et al.*, 1999; Roughead *et al.*, 2003; Zwart *et al.*, 2005). However, in one of them, the authors report an increase of hydroxyproline (a bone resorption marker) that could be related to the protein source: a collagen-rich meat (Roughead *et al.*, 2003). On the other hand, three studies considering both formation and resorption markers concluded that there was a positive effect of protein on bone. One of them observed a decrease of desoxypyridinoline (a bone resorption marker) with stable formation, indicating a positive decoupling (Hunt *et al.*, 2009). In the second study, both formation and resorption markers increased in a protein-supplemented group compared to control during 6 months of exercise. According to the authors, bone formation will increase faster than bone resorption over time (Ballard *et al.*, 2005). In the final study, a one year soy protein supplementation only increased bone formation markers while resorption markers remained at the same level (Arjmandi *et al.*, 2005). Finally, two intervention studies reported a decrease of resorption with protein supplementation but provided no data on bone formation (Dawson-Hughes *et al.*, 2004; Ince *et al.*, 2004).

3. Protein and calcium metabolism

3.1 Urine calcium

Urinary calcium excretion is the major pathway for body calcium loss, along with that of feces and sweat. A high urinary calcium level has been linked to increased bone loss (Giannini *et al.*, 2003).

Numerous studies have reported a positive linear relationship between dietary protein and urinary calcium (Kerstetter & Allen, 1990; Kerstetter *et al.*, 2003; Whiting *et al.*, 1997). The rise in urinary calcium with protein intake has also been observed in more recent studies (Ceglia *et al.*, 2009; Hunt *et al.*, 2009; Jajoo *et al.*, 2006). In one study, no effect of protein on calciuria was observed (Roughead *et al.*, 2003). The mechanism underlying the effect of protein on calcium excretion is debated. First, a high protein diet induces an increase of glomerular filtration rate which will exacerbate any increased calcium excretion (Kerstetter *et al.*, 1998). According to the acid ash hypothesis, the calciuric effect of a high protein intake would be caused by the protein-induced acid load. A meta-analysis by Fenton *et al.* of over 25 studies concluded that changes in acid excretion modulate calcium excretion (Fenton *et al.*, 2008). Other studies showed that urinary calcium could be reduced by decreasing the acid load (L. Frassetto *et al.*, 2005; Lemann *et al.*, 1991). The systemic acidosis generated by the protein load inhibits TRPV5 calcium channel expression in the kidney. Because TRPV5 participates in renal calcium reabsorption, its inhibition increases urinary calcium (Nijenhuis *et al.*, 2006).

Another mechanism for the protein-induced calcium excretion was proposed by Conigrave and colleagues, involving the extracellular CaSR (Conigrave *et al.*, 2008). CaSR found on cells of the parathyroid glands and in the renal tubules are sensitive not only to calcium, but also to some AAs (Conigrave *et al.*, 2000). Through this double sensitivity, a link is formed between protein and calcium metabolism. According to these findings, AAs would activate the CaSRs, reducing parathormone (PTH) production and decreasing renal calcium reabsorption, leading eventually to an increased calcium excretion (Conigrave *et al.*, 2008). Indeed, PTH level has been shown to be influenced by protein intake (Kerstetter *et al.*, 1997, 1998, 2006).

Urinary calcium loss due to a high protein diet was attributed to enhanced bone resorption (Kerstetter & Allen, 1990); however, this view has been discussed as the link between protein and bone resorption is unclear (Bonjour, 2005; M. Thorpe & Evans, 2011). Urinary calcium excretion is mainly related to bone as the main calcium storage compartment. However, an increase of the excreted calcium could also be related to an increase in calcium absorption through the diet. Hence the effect of protein on intestinal calcium absorption should also be considered.

3.2 Calcium absorption

While many studies claim that high-protein diets cause calciuria, there is no clear relationship between protein intake and calcium absorption. Some studies report a positive effect of protein on calcium absorption (Cao *et al.*, 2011; Hunt *et al.*, 2009; Kerstetter *et al.*, 1998, 2005). One study of 13 women observed an increase in calcium absorption that explained 93% of the calcium excretion (Kerstetter *et al.*, 2005). Another study reported an increased calciuria and a non-significant increase in calcium absorption with protein intake. But the net difference between calcium absorption and excretion with high or low protein intake remained stable (Cao *et al.*, 2011). However, other studies observed a decrease of calcium absorption with protein (Dawson-Hughes & Harris, 2002; Heaney, 2000), or no effect at all (Roughead *et al.*, 2003). It should be pointed out that all studies showing a positive effect were short term studies (2 to 7 weeks) whereas the two studies with a negative effect were long-term studies (years). It is thus possible that protein increases calcium absorption at first and that this effect is reversed in the long run.

The effect of protein on calcium absorption could also be conditioned by the calcium intake itself. Two studies tested the effect of protein intake on intestinal calcium absorption at different levels of calcium intake. One observed a positive effect of protein for 675 mg Ca/d and no effect at 1510 mg Ca/d (Hunt *et al.*, 2009) whereas an other study observed a negative effect at 871 mg/d and no effect at 1346 mg/d.

Moreover, Kerstetter et al. repeatedly showed that, in the context of low protein intake, there is both an increase of PTH and a decrease in calcium absorption (Kerstetter *et al.*, 1997, 1998, 2006). Those two findings seem incompatible because PTH is known to increase calcium absorption (Heaney, 2007). However, Conigrave *et al.*, as a part of his theory on amino acid-sensing CaSR, proposes another mechanism not involving PTH. CaSR is also present in the gastro-intestinal tract, where it promotes gastric acid secretion directly and indirectly through gastrin release (Conigrave & Brown, 2006). High-protein diets induce the acidification of the intestinal content which helps calcium salts to dissolve into Ca^{2+}, thereby facilitating its absorption even if PTH level is low (Conigrave *et al.*, 2008).

3.3 The acid-ash theory

According to the acid-ash theory, some foods such as protein would induce a metabolic acidosis whereas other foods such as vegetables and fruits would counteract this process. The acidosis resulting from a high protein diet would be deleterious to bone and induce bone loss.

Dietary proteins, and more specifically their sulphur AA content, are part of the acid-forming nutrients. Consequently, high protein consumption would lead to metabolic acidosis (Frassetto *et al.*, 1998; Kerstetter *et al.*, 2006). pH is closely regulated in the body and any increase of the acid load is buffered through different pathways. The main one is through lung excretion of CO_2, followed by kidney acid excretion. Bone has also been proposed to take part by releasing Ca^{2+} (Lemann *et al.*, 2003). This last pathway is debated because the lungs' and the kidneys' buffering capacity are considered to be sufficient to compensate for the protein-induced acidosis (Bonjour, 2005). The idea that an acidic diet is deleterious for bone is supported by observational studies linking acid production to a reduced BMD (New *et al.*, 2004; Rahbar *et al.*, 2009; Wynn *et al.*, 2008). Intervention studies on this topic usually correct the acid diet of the subjects by supplementing them with alkalinizing molecules. The results consistently show an improvement of bone health with the supplementation. This improvement occurs at the level of urinary calcium excretion (Frassetto *et al.*, 2005; Lemann *et al.*, 1991), bone turnover markers (Dawson-Hughes *et al.*, 2009; He *et al.*, 2010; Maurer *et al.*, 2003) or Bone Mineral Density (BMD) (Domrongkitchaiporn *et al.*, 2002). Despite all this evidence of the beneficial effect of alkalinizing the diet, it should be noted that according to a recent meta-analysis, no causal link could be established between dietary acid load and bone disease (Fenton *et al.*, 2011). It is also important to consider that the findings supporting the acid-ash hypothesis are based on an alkalinisation of the diet and are not directly related to protein intake.

A decrease of pH is probably one of the main activators of bone-resorbing osteoclasts and an inhibitor of bone matrix deposition by osteoblasts, which explains the acid-induced bone reabsorption (Arnett, 2008). Extrapolation of these results to the clinical level is risky as it compares the *in vitro* pH variation to a high protein-induced acidosis. Indeed, the pH variation induced by protein intake is likely to be too small to induce any effect in the bone micro-environment (Bonjour, 2005).

Although they lead to different conclusions, the acid-ash theory and the hormonal anabolic theory are not mutually exclusive. A dual-pathway model for the effect of protein on bone has been proposed (M. Thorpe & Evans, 2011). Although it has been recently criticized in a meta-analysis (Fenton *et al.*, 2011), it seems that there is a beneficial effect of diet alkalinisation. This can be achieved by lowering acidic or by increasing alkaline food consumption. When considering protein, the second method is more beneficial. Indeed, even if protein is an acid nutrient, it is also an activator of bone anabolic hormones and its consumption should not be lowered. This is especially true in populations already consuming a low protein diet such as the elderly. The acid load resulting from the protein consumption should be compensated by an increased consumption of alkalinizing fruits and vegetables.

Some diets designed to promote weight loss rely on high protein consumption for a quick effect on weight. It is hard to estimate what is the effect of such diets on bone. Indeed, hyperproteic diets imply also potentially confounding effect such as spontaneous caloric restriction and a possible lack of micronutrients. Moreover, the wide variety of hyperproteic diets and the potential lack of compliance of the subjects further increase the difficulty of designing an adequate study on the subject.

4. Protein and bone parameters

4.1 Bone Mineral Density

BMD is not the only determinant of skeletal fragility; the spatial distribution of the bone mass (as cortical and trabecular bone) and the intrinsic material properties of bone are also major components (Bouxsein & Seeman, 2009). Measuring BMD or Bone Mineral Content (BMC) is the easiest way of directly assessing bone strength in humans.

Most observation studies report a positive association between protein and bone density (Hannan *et al.*, 2000; Promislow *et al.*, 2002) or between protein and BMD change (Dawson-Hughes & Harris, 2002; Vatanparast *et al.*, 2007). Specific studies showing a positive correlation between protein and bone density cover a broad population: premenopausal women (Teegarden *et al.*, 1998), postmenopausal women (Devine *et al.*, 2005; Ilich *et al.*, 2003; Rapuri *et al.*, 2003; M. Thorpe *et al.*, 2008b), men (Whiting *et al.*, 2002) and children (Alexy *et al.*, 2005; Chevalley *et al.*, 2008).

On the other hand, two studies on premenopausal women concluded that protein intake had no relation with BMD (Beasley *et al.*, 2010; Mazess & Barden, 1991). One study reported a negative association with BMC (Metz *et al.*, 1993). Finally, a case-control study compared 134 osteoporotic women with 137 controls and identified total protein intake as a risk factor for osteoporosis. A meta-analysis by Darling and colleagues conclude that there is no evidence of a negative effect of protein intake on bone when looking at observation studies; in fact there is probably a small positive effect of protein on bone (Darling *et al.*, 2009).

There are very few interventional studies comparing high vs. low protein intake. One of them focused on the effect of an AA and carbohydrate supplement during bed rest on 13 men. The study lasted 28 days and the authors reported a decrease in BMC in the supplemented subjects whereas BMC in control subjects remained stable (Zwart *et al.*, 2005). It should be noted that energy intake was different between the two groups due to an energy-free placebo. Another study supplemented hospitalized elderly men and women for 38 days with 20.4g of protein. Along with other positive effects (lower complication rate, shorter hospital stay), the authors reported a decrease in BMD loss with the protein supplement (Tkatch *et al.*, 1992). Finally, a year-long study supplementing 62 postmenopausal women with 25g of soy protein observed no effect on total hip BMD or BMC (Arjmandi *et al.*, 2005).

4.2 Fracture risk

Fracture risk is the ultimate clinical outcome when considering bone. A longitudinal study of 32 050 postmenopausal women observed a reduced relative risk of hip fracture when protein intake was increased (Munger *et al.*, 1999). Another one observed that a reduction in wrist fracture is positively associated with the consumption frequency of high protein food in 1865 perimenopausal women (D. L. Thorpe *et al.*, 2008a). Finally, in a case-control study on 1167 cases of hip fractures and 1334 controls of both sexes aged 50-89, the odds ratio for hip fracture decreased with the increase of protein intake (Wengreen *et al.*, 2004).

According to these three studies, protein would have a beneficial effect on bone, but some other studies found conflicting results (Dargent-Molina *et al.*, 2008; Feskanich *et al.*, 1996; Meyer *et al.*, 1997). However, it should be noted that the negative relationship between protein and fracture risk was significant only in the lowest quartiles of calcium intake (<400 mg/d) and that no association was observed for higher calcium intake (Dargent-Molina *et al.*, 2008; Meyer *et al.*, 1997). Pooling four studies in a meta-analysis, Darling found no significant effect of protein on the risk ratio of fracture (Darling *et al.*, 2009). To our knowledge, it seems that as long as calcium intake is sufficient there is a protective effect of protein on bone that lowers the fracture risk.

The question of the effect of protein on fracture healing has also been addressed in some randomised controlled trials. All four trials were conducted by the same group and reported that a protein supplement improved the patients' condition after a low-trauma femoral neck fracture (Delmi *et al.*, 1990; Tkatch *et al.*, 1992) or hip fracture (Chevalley *et al.*, 2008; Schurch *et al.*, 1998). All the clinical trials had very similar design: patients were about 80 years old and the protein supplement given was 20g. According to the two studies on femoral neck fracture, patients taking the protein supplementation had better clinical outcomes and reduced rate of complication and mortality during the hospital stay and 6 months after (Delmi *et al.*, 1990; Tkatch *et al.*, 1992). After hip fracture, the protein supplement increased IGF-1, attenuating bone loss at 6 months and shortening hospital stay (Schurch *et al.*, 1998). The IGF-1 increase is independent of the type of protein given (casein, whey protein or whey protein and amino acids) (Chevalley *et al.*, 2010). The beneficial effect of protein is probably linked to both the increased IGF-1 level and the correction of the patient nutritional state.

5. Effect of specific protein source on bone

Each protein bares some information in the form of its chain of amino acids. This information can relate to specific effects of some proteins. When protein goes through the intestinal barrier, 50% are completely degraded as simple amino acids, 40% are partly degraded as peptides and 10% remain intact (Mallegol *et al.*, 2005). This observation means that half of the digested protein reaching blood is still bearing some information in the form of the AA chain. Much research has tried to investigate what might be the best source of protein for bone health.

5.1 Animal vs. vegetable protein

Some observational studies considered the nature of protein source when measuring the effect on bone. One of them studied the relationships between the animal/vegetable protein ratio and bone parameters on 1035 postmenopausal women, showing that the ratio is positively associated with bone loss and hip fracture risk (Sellmeyer *et al.*, 2001). However, the fact that a ratio was used in this study instead of the absolute values has been criticized (Bonjour, 2005; M. Thorpe & Evans, 2011). Other observational studies provide conflicting results. BMD was positively associated with animal protein intake and negatively to vegetable intake in one study (Promislow *et al.*, 2002) but the opposite association was found when considering bone ultrasound attenuation (Weikert *et al.*, 2005). Low levels of both protein types have been associated with deleterious effects on bone: low animal protein is related to bone loss (Hannan *et al.*, 2000) and low vegetable protein is related to low BMD (Beasley *et al.*, 2010). These results suggest that a minimum intake of both proteins is required regardless of the source. Finally, when considering fracture risk, a positive relationship was found with both animal (Dargent-Molina *et al.*, 2008; Feskanich *et al.*, 1996; Meyer *et al.*, 1997) and vegetable protein (Munger *et al.*, 1999; D. L. Thorpe *et al.*, 2008a). It should be noted that the studies finding a positive relationship between animal protein and fracture risk also found a positive relationship with total protein. On the other hand, those finding a positive relationship between vegetable protein and fracture risk reported a negative one with total protein. Hence the results for animal and vegetable protein are not obtained in the same context.

The intervention studies comparing animal and vegetable protein always focus on specific types of protein, usually soy and casein. Hence it is the specific effect of those proteins that is evaluated and not the one of the animal and vegetable food groups. The only whole-diet intervention study was based on meat or protein-rich vegetables such as nuts and grains. Only urinary parameters were measured and urinary calcium was similar for the two diets (Massey & Kynast-Gales, 2001). More studies of this type are needed to address this issue.

Mechanistically, the reason for differentiating animal from vegetable protein is their differing sulphur AA content and the consequent modulation of potential acid load (Sellmeyer *et al.*, 2001). The influence of sulphate content on protein efficiency has been emphasized in a cross-sectional study on 161 postmenopausal women. The results show a positive association of total protein intake with lumbar spine and total hip BMD; however, in lumbar spine this benefit is suppressed by the sulphur-containing AAs (M. Thorpe *et al.*, 2008b). The authors conclude that an excessive consumption of sulphur AAs is likely to be deleterious for bone. However, as underlined by Massey, the assumption that animal protein contains more sulphur AA than vegetable protein is not always true. As an example, potential acidity from sulphur AA in milk or beef is lower than that of whole wheat or white rice (Massey, 2003). Hence, even if sulphur AAs were proven to have a negative effect on bone, the extrapolation to animal and vegetable food groups is likely to give incorrect results because of the broad variety of foods in these groups. In future research, it would be more accurate to consider an estimation of the sulphate content of each protein-containing food rather than focusing only on a crude animal-vegetable distinction.

5.2 Milk proteins

Milk contains many bioactive factors, including growth hormones, enzymes, antimicrobials, anti-inflammatory agents, transporters and peptide or nonpeptide hormones. Milk, because it contains bioactive molecules, extends beyond applications in infant nutrition and was considered as a possible source of factors with anabolic effects on bone.

5.2.1 Milk Basic Proteins (MBP)

Clinical trials showed that MBP supplementation increased BMD and decreased bone resorption biomarkers in healthy women (Aoe *et al.*, 2001; Uenishi *et al.*, 2007; Yamamura *et al.*, 2002), menopausal women (Aoe *et al.*, 2005), and healthy older women (Aoyagi *et al.*, 2010). In particular, MBP suppresses osteoclast-mediated bone resorption and leads to reduced osteoclast number in animal studies (Morita *et al.*, 2008). Morita *et al.* reported that the protein fraction responsible for the observed activities of MBP is the bovine angiogenin which acts as a bone resorption-inhibitory protein (Morita *et al.*, 2008).

However, not all studies have shown a beneficial effect of MBP. In one study, 84 healthy young women were divided into three groups receiving placebo, whole milk, or milk containing 40 mg MBP for 8 months. Compared with the baseline values, total BMD significantly increased in all groups. There was a significant decrease of bone resorption marker N-teleopeptides of type-I collagen (NTx) while bone formation remained stable in both milk groups. (Zou *et al.*, 2009).

HPLC analysis of the major proteins in the MBP fraction identified the presence of the glycoprotein lactoferrin in most of these fractions (Naot *et al.*, 2005).

5.2.2 Lactoferrin

Lactoferrin (LF) is an 80 kDa iron-binding glycoprotein of the transferrin family. This molecule has been demonstrated to inhibit *in vitro* osteoclast-mediated bone resorption (Lorget *et al.*, 2002). LF was also demonstrated to have *in vitro* anabolic, differentiating and anti-apoptotic effects on osteoblasts, and to inhibit osteoclastogenesis. Moreover *in vivo* local injection of LF above the hemicalvaria increases bone formation and bone area in adult mice (Cornish *et al.*, 2004). LF has a role in host non-specific defense (Gahr *et al.*, 1991; Legrand *et al.*, 2004). In addition to its direct antimicrobial effects, LF is believed to modulate the inflammatory process mainly by preventing the release of inflammatory cytokines which induce recruitment and activation of immune cells at inflammatory sites (Legrand *et al.*, 2005).

Investigations of our group and others established that LF at physiological concentrations can stimulate proliferation of primary osteoblasts and osteoblastic-cell lines and increase osteoblast differentiation (Blais *et al.*, 2009; Cornish, 2004; Takayama & Mizumachi, 2008). Studies using 3-week culture of primary rat osteoblasts show that LF dose-dependently increases the number of nodules and the area of mineralized bone formed (Cornish, 2004). Our *in vitro* experiments demonstrated that LF could directly act on bone cells. Bovine LF (bLF) at low physiological concentrations (5 µg/ml) stimulates growth and activity of osteoblastic MC3T3-E1 cells and primary culture of murine osteoblast bone cells (Blais *et al.*, 2009). Low density lipoprotein receptor-related protein 1 and 2, which are present on osteoblastic cells, have been shown to be partially responsible for LF's mitogenic effect in osteoblasts (Grey *et al.*, 2004). Moreover, Grey *et al.*, showed that LF is able to protect osteoblastic cells from apoptosis induced by serum withdrawal (Grey *et al.*, 2006).

LF action on osteoclasts is strikingly different since it produces an important arrest of osteoclastogenesis (Cornish, 2004; Lorget *et al.*, 2002). However, LF does not modulate mature ostoeclast activity. bLF at a concentration ranging from 10 to 1000 µg/ml was found to inhibit pre-osteoclastic established RAW cell growth. These results were confirmed in mixed primary culture of murine bone cells (Blais *et al.*, 2009). In contrast, there was no effect of LF on bone resorption when tested on isolated mature osteoclasts, or in organ cultures that can detect mature osteoclast activity (Grey *et al.*, 2006).

In vivo bone effects of LF were first studied using local injection of LF above the hemicalvaria which increased bone formation and bone area in adult mice (Cornish, 2004). Few recent studies using ovariectomized (OVX) rodents as a model for post menopausal bone loss measured the effect of dietary supplementation on bone (Blais *et al.*, 2009; Guo *et al.*, 2009; Malet *et al.*, 2011). LF administered orally to OVX rats for three months protected them against the OVX-induced reduction of bone volume and BMD and increased the parameters of mechanical strength, increased bone formation and reduced bone resorption (Guo *et al.*, 2009). Our studies using OVX mice demonstrated that the dietary bLF transfer into peripheral blood. LF supplementation increases BMD and bone strength compared to the OVX control group. This study supports a direct effect of LF on bone cells (Blais *et al.*, 2009).

Recent animal studies demonstrated that estrogen deficiency causes bone loss by mechanisms associated with inflammatory and oxidative processes (Grassi *et al.*, 2007; Lean *et al.*, 2003; Muthusami *et al.*, 2005). TNFα is one of the cytokines responsible for the augmented osteoclastogenesis (Suda *et al.*, 1999). Indeed, ovariectomy causes an increase in TNF production from T-cells which in turn increases macrophage colony-stimulating factor and RANKL levels, leading to osteoclastogenesis (Cornish *et al.*, 2004; Suda *et al.*, 1999). Moreover the presence of increased levels of TNFα was reported in the bone marrow of OVX animals and in blood cells of postmenopausal women (Oh *et al.*, 2007; Shanker *et al.*, 1994). Postmenopausal osteoporosis should also be regarded as the result of an inflammatory process (Weitzmann & Pacifici, 2007). It has been shown that bLF plays a role in host non-specific defense and modulates the inflammatory process mainly by preventing the release of inflammatory cytokines that induce recruitment and activation of immune cells at inflammatory sites (Debbabi *et al.*, 1998; Legrand *et al.*, 2006). Indeed, bLF enriched diet ingestion can reduce release of pro-inflammatory cytokines and increase anti-inflammatory cytokine production. Our studies showed that bLF ingestion decreases bone loss and bone resorption markers. A decreased TNFα mRNA expression associated with a TNFα production inhibition on peripheral T-lymphocytes was observed with a bLF supplementation in OVX mice. Furthermore, bLF can prevent lymphocyte activation and cytokine release in the bone micro-environment. Production and release of TNFα were strongly down-regulated by LF. These immune modulations were spatially and temporally correlated with reduced bone loss. We suggested that bLF modulates the inflammatory process via specific TNFα inhibition in order to improve bone loss (Malet *et al.*, 2011). Recently a clinical trial of 38 healthy postmenopausal women randomized into placebo or ribonuclease-enriched-LF (R-ELF) groups evaluated bone health status over a period of 12 months. The authors demonstrated that R-ELF supplementation reduced bone resorption and increased osteoblastic bone formation; however BMD was not evaluated (Bharadwaj *et al.*, 2009).

In conclusion, LF has a positive effect on bone health and might be useful in pathological states of reduced bone density. The molecular mechanisms are not fully understood but our studies suggest that dietary bLF supplementation can have a beneficial effect on postmenopausal bone loss not only via a direct effect but also by modulating immune function. The development of pharmaceutical or nutriceutical compounds that are based on LF will require a better understanding of LF's mechanism of action on bone.

5.3 Collagen

Collagen has a unique triple helix configuration with a repeating sequence $(Gly\text{-}X\text{-}Y)_n$, with X and Y being mostly proline and hydroxyproline (Hyp) (Bos *et al.*, 1999; Ramshaw *et al.*, 1998). Some studies suggest that a hydrolyzed collagen-enriched diet improves bone collagen metabolism and BMD. Oral administration of Hydrolyzed Collagen (HC) increased BMC and BMD in rats and mice fed a calcium or protein deficient diet (Koyama *et al.*, 2001; Wu *et al.*, 2004).

5.3.1 Ingestion of collagen

Oral administration of HC was demonstrated to increase the quantity of type I collagen and proteoglycans in the bone matrix of ovariectomized rats (Nomura *et al.*, 2005). Moreover, in patients with osteoporosis, oral intake of HC with calcitonin had a stronger inhibitory effect on bone resorption than calcitonin alone (Adam *et al.*, 1996). Oesser *et al.* demonstrated the intestinal absorption and cartilage accumulation of collagen-derived peptides (Oesser *et al.*, 1999). It has been generally assumed that collagen-rich diets interact with the bone matrix. Indeed, collagen-derived di- and tripeptides rich in hydroxyproline such as Hyp, Pro-Hyp, Pro-Hyp-Gly or Gly-Pro-Val have been detected in human blood following the ingestion of HC (Iwai *et al.*, 2005). The PEPT1 proton-dependent transporter assures the transport of Pro-Hyp across the intestinal barrier (Aito-Inoue *et al.*, 2007).

A study of Ohara *et al.* compared quantity and structures of food-derived gelatin hydrolysates in human blood from fish scale, fish skin and pork skin type I collagen in a single blind crossover study (Ohara *et al.*, 2007). Amounts of free Hyp and Hyp-containing peptide were measured over a 24-h period. Hyp-containing peptides comprised approximately 30% of all detected Hyp. However, efficiency of HC ingestion depends not only on collagen origin but also on the molecular size of the HC. Collagen needs to be hydrolysed to be able to interact with bone metabolism.

5.3.2 *In vivo* studies

Our *in vivo* studies indicate that ingestion of HC diet induced the growth of the external diameter of the bone cortical zone in OVX mice (Guillerminet *et al.*, 2010, 2011). The increased cortical area was correlated with a significant increase in the femur external diameter, without modification of the size of the medullar area. Therefore, the increased size of the cortical area was induced by a periosteal apposition of bone on the mouse femur. Due to this increase in bone size, the ultimate strength of femurs of OVX-mice ingesting HC was significantly greater than the control OVX mice. The increase of the external diameter was also related to a higher level of bone ALP during the first month of HC ingestion. However, the effect was transient; after three months no significant ALP increase was reported. Moreover, HC ingestion was able to increase the bone non-mineral content. There was no significant modification of Young's modulus but bone stiffness increased. Assuming that the stiffness of bone is correlated to the amount of type I collagen present (Burr, 2002; Mann *et al.*, 2001), and since some previous studies showed an increase of type I collagen and proteoglycan excretion for mice fed hydrolyzed collagen, we can propose that HC ingestion increases type I collagen formation in mouse bone.

5.3.3 *In vitro* studies

The *in vitro* results obtained with primary tissue culture of murine bone cells confirmed that HC was able to stimulate cell growth and ALP activity. In our studies, all the tested collagens were able to increase osteoblast activity but the 2kDA porcine HC was the most efficient *in vitro* (Guillerminet *et al.*, 2010). Similar observations were also reported with osteoblasts grown on collagen type I films compared to a plastic support with an improvement in various bone markers including increased ALP activity and an accelerated and uniform mineralization of the bone matrix (Lynch *et al.*, 1995). Moreover, our work using the *in vitro* BD BioCoat™ Osteologic™ bone cell culture system showed that PCH-N hydrolyzed collagen did not modify osteoclast growth but reduced osteoclast differentiation (Guillerminet *et al.*, 2010). This effect, combined with increased osteoblast activity is likely to modulate bone turnover leading to the growth of the external diameter of cortical bone.

5.3.4 Mechanism of action

Several potential mechanisms can be proposed to explain the influence of HC-derived peptides on bone metabolism. Some results have suggested that ingestion of type I hydrolyzed collagen leads to the production and absorption of collagen-derived peptides similar to peptides released from type I collagen *in situ* during bone resorption. Those peptides also act on bone cell metabolism (Adam *et al.*, 1996). Osteoblast activity involves three steps including proliferation, matrix protein synthesis (type I collagen and proteoglycans) and mineralization of the bone matrix (Owen *et al.*, 1991; Quarles *et al.*, 1992; Stein & Lian, 1993). Several hormones and cytokines can modulate osteoblast and osteoclast differentiation and activity. The cytokine TGF-β which is stored in a latent form in the bone matrix, and secreted during the bone resorption phase, is believed to exert such an effect (Oreffo *et al.*, 1989). TGF-β stimulates type I collagen and proteoglycan production while inhibiting that of hydroxyapatite. Interestingly, the type I collagen-derived peptide DGEA (asparagine, glycine, glutamine and alanine), was shown to interact with $\alpha 2\beta 1$ integrin located on the osteoblast cell membrane. This interaction leads to inhibition of TGF-β and consequently bone matrix protein synthesis (Oesser *et al.*, 1999; Takeuchi *et al.*, 1996, 1997; Xiao *et al.*, 1998). Moreover, Hyp is an aromatic AA, and an increase of its concentration can, as suggested previously, increase IGF-1 levels which consequently attenuates bone loss.

Taken together, the results indicate that hydrolyzed collagen modulates bone formation and mineralization of the bone matrix by stimulating osteoblast growth and differentiation while reducing osteoclast differentiation. These effects lead to growth of the external diameter of the cortical zone.

5.4 Isoflavone-containing soy protein

Soy contains isoflavones able to bind to estrogen receptors (Folman & Pope, 1969). They have received considerable interest as a possible alternative to conventional Hormone Replacement Therapy (HRT). However, the efficiency of phytoestrogens such as soy isoflavone on bone is still to be proven.

Epidemiological studies suggest that populations with high soy intake (such as Asian populations) have a lower incidence of osteoporotic fractures (Adlercreutz & Mazur, 1997; Schwartz *et al.*, 1999). Asian women typically consume about 20g of soy daily which provides 40 mg of isoflavones (Chen *et al.*, 1999; Ho *et al.*, 2003). However, lower rates of fracture in these populations may not be fully attributed to soy consumption as ethnic related variation in fracture rates can also be explained by differences in bone structure (Bouxsein, 2011).

Many animal studies show that soy protein and/or its isoflavones have positive effects on bone mineral density (BMD) (Arjmandi *et al.*, 1998a, 1998b). However, clinical trial results ranged from no significant changes (Alekel *et al.*, 2000; Dalais *et al.*, 1998; Gallagher *et al.*, 2004; Kreijkamp-Kaspers *et al.*, 2004; Potter *et al.*, 1998) to a slight increase (Chiechi *et al.*, 2002; Lydeking-Olsen *et al.*, 2004; Potter *et al.*, 1998) in BMD. The bone protective effects of soy and/or its isoflavones are at best inconclusive.

5.4.1 Types of isoflavones

The major isoflavones in soy foods include genistein and diadzein. Genistein 2 has one-third of the potency of estradiol 1 when it interacts with estrogen receptor-b (ER-b), and one-thousandth of the potency of estradiol 1 when it interacts with ER-a. Hence Genistein 2 can induce a small estradiol-like response in bone tissues (Adlercreutz & Mazur, 1997; Zhou *et al.*, 2003). Another isoflavone, called equol, is not present in soybean but is a metabolic product of the biotransformation of diadzein by gut bacteria (Setchell *et al.*, 2002). 80% of the Asian population are equol producers (Fujimoto *et al.*, 2008; Morton *et al.*, 2002). In contrast, as few as 25% of individuals in North America and Europe are able to make S-equol (Lampe *et al.*, 1998).

5.4.2 Isoflavone and bone fracture

A number of reviews describe the effects of dietary soy and isoflavones on bone (Jackson *et al.*, 2011; Messina, 2010; Reinwald & Weaver, 2010). Among the studies exploring the effect of isoflavone-containing food on BMD in postmenopausal women, few report a relationship between soy consumption and the risk of bone fracture. A clinical trial conducted by Marini *et al.* found that in postmenopausal osteopenic Italians receiving 54mg/day genistein for two years, spinal BMD increased by 5.8% (n=150), whereas it decreased in the placebo group by 6.3% (n=154). Similar effects were reported for the hip (Marini *et al.*, 2007). However, recently published long-term trials do not confirm these results; only the trial conducted by Alekel *et al.* reports a modest effect at the femoral neck with 120mg/d isoflavone but no effect with 80mg/d (Alekel *et al.*, 2009).

In contrast clinical trials investigating associations between soy-food intake and BMD in Japanese or Chinese healthy postmenopausal women report that higher isoflavone consumption is associated with lower risk of bone fracture (Ho *et al.*, 2003; Ikeda *et al.*, 2006; Kaneki *et al.*, 2001). Analysis of fracture incidence in the Shanghai cohort (Zhang *et al.*, 2005) and of hip fracture in the Singapore cohort (Koh *et al.*, 2009) shows in both studies one-third reductions in fracture risk when comparing high- with low-soy consumers.

5.4.3 Factors modulating the effect of soy on bone health

The effectiveness of dietary adaptation of western populations which rarely consumed soy must be considered. East Asian participants in epidemiological studies did not require an adaptation period or an interruption of life-long dietary habits like a western population would. Hence the observation cannot be extrapolated from one population to another.

It may be less difficult to determine bone effects following a life-long intake of traditional foods compared with intermittent intakes of soy. Traditional soy foods are a complex blend of isoflavones, protein, lipids, vitamins, minerals and other bioactive compounds that may act individually and/or synergistically to exert healthy effects. Supplements included in western diets provide quantities of individual soy components. Types of whole soy food consumed (fermented vs. nonfermented) and/or ethnicity (equol producers) may also affect outcome interpretation of soy bone effects.

Long-term observational studies in Asian populations support a benefit of traditional soy food consumption on bone health in this population. The health effects of soy-bean phytoestrogens in non-Asian postmenopausal women are promising. No conclusive evidence supports that the isoflavones from the sources studied do have beneficial effects on bone health. More researches are needed to clarify the role of dietary phytoestrogen in osteoporosis prevention.

6. Conclusion

Protein acts on bone metabolism at different levels and through different mechanisms. There is little evidence that a high-protein diet will increase bone loss. Protein is well-known to be calciuric, yet there are conflicting data on whether the excreted calcium comes from an increase of calcium absorption or from bone resorption. The direct effects of protein on bone turnover markers and BMD seem to be positive when considering observational studies, but interventional studies do not provide significant outcomes to conclude. Finally, when considering fracture rate, there seems to be a small positive effect of protein on bone as long as calcium levels remain adequate.

Two mechanisms are proposed to explain the action of protein on bone: the acid-ash theory and the hormonal anabolic effect through IGF-1 and CaSR. The hormonal anabolic mechanism supports the fact that protein is beneficial to bone by increasing IGF-1. On the other hand, the acid-ash theory considers that the acid load due to protein consumption is harmful to bone. If both mechanisms occur at the same time, it is possible to benefit from the protein-induced IGF-1 without the negative effect of the acid load by compensating the diet with adequate alkalinizing foods.

Dietary protein quality adds complexity to the protein debate. It has been hypothesized that animal protein would be more deleterious to bone than vegetal protein. However, studies show no real difference between those two protein sources. Similarly, long-term observational studies support a benefit of traditional soy food consumption on bone health, but no conclusive evidence supports the hypothesis that this is due to the isoflavones. On the other hand, some peptides obtained from protein digestion have been shown to be helpful to prevent bone loss. Recent results indicate that HC could be of potential interest for nutritional intervention in the prevention of bone loss. Moreover, LF has been reported to have a positive effect on bone health and might be useful in pathological states of reduced bone density. The molecular mechanisms are not fully understood but our studies suggest that dietary bLF supplementation can have a beneficial effect on postmenopausal bone loss not only by acting on bone cells but also by modulating immune function.

7. References

Adam, M.; Spacek, P.; Hulejova, H.; Galianova, A. & Blahos, J. (1996). [Postmenopausal osteoporosis. Treatment with calcitonin and a diet rich in collagen proteins]. *Cas Lek Cesk*, Vol. 135, No. 3, (Jan 31 1996), pp. 74-78

Adlercreutz, H. & Mazur, W. (1997). Phyto-oestrogens and Western diseases. *Ann Med*, Vol. 29, No. 2, (Apr 1997), pp. 95-120

Aito-Inoue, M.; Lackeyram, D.; Fan, M.Z.; Sato, K. & Mine, Y. (2007). Transport of a tripeptide, Gly-Pro-Hyp, across the porcine intestinal brush-border membrane. *J Pept Sci*, Vol. 13, No. 7, (Jul 2007), pp. 468-474

Alekel, D.L.; Germain, A.S.; Peterson, C.T.; Hanson, K.B.; Stewart, J.W. & Toda, T. (2000). Isoflavone-rich soy protein isolate attenuates bone loss in the lumbar spine of perimenopausal women. *Am J Clin Nutr*, Vol. 72, No. 3, (Sep 2000), pp. 844-852

Alekel, D.L.; Van Loan, M.D.; Koehler, K.J.; Hanson, L.N.; Stewart, J.W.; Hanson, K.B.; Kurzer, M.S. & Peterson, C.T. (2009). The soy isoflavones for reducing bone loss (SIRBL) study: a 3-y randomized controlled trial in postmenopausal women. *Am J Clin Nutr*, Vol. 91, No. 1, (Jan 2009), pp. 218-230

Alexy, U.; Remer, T.; Manz, F.; Neu, C.M. & Schoenau, E. (2005). Long-term protein intake and dietary potential renal acid load are associated with bone modeling and remodeling at the proximal radius in healthy children. *Am J Clin Nutr*, Vol. 82, No. 5, (Nov 2005), pp. 1107-1114

Aoe, S.; Koyama, T.; Toba, Y.; Itabashi, A. & Takada, Y. (2005). A controlled trial of the effect of milk basic protein (MBP) supplementation on bone metabolism in healthy menopausal women. *Osteoporos Int*, Vol. 16, No. 12, (Dec 2005), pp. 2123-2128

Aoe, S.; Toba, Y.; Yamamura, J.; Kawakami, H.; Yahiro, M.; Kumegawa, M.; Itabashi, A. & Takada, Y. (2001). Controlled trial of the effects of milk basic protein (MBP) supplementation on bone metabolism in healthy adult women. *Biosci Biotechnol Biochem*, Vol. 65, No. 4, (Apr 2001), pp. 913-918

Aoyagi, Y.; Park, H.; Park, S.; Yoshiuchi, K.; Kikuchi, H.; Kawakami, H.; Morita, Y.; Ono, A. & Shephard RJ (2010). Interactive effects of milk basic protein supplements and habitual physical activity on bone health in older women: A 1-year randomized controlled trial. *Int Dairy J*, Vol. 20, No. (Mar 2010), pp. 724-730

Arjmandi, B.H.; Birnbaum, R.; Goyal, N.V.; Getlinger, M.J.; Juma, S.; Alekel, L.; Hasler, C.M.; Drum, M.L.; Hollis, B.W. & Kukreja, S.C. (1998a). Bone-sparing effect of soy protein in ovarian hormone-deficient rats is related to its isoflavone content. *Am J Clin Nutr*, Vol. 68, No. 6 Suppl, (Dec 1998a), pp. 1364S-1368S

Arjmandi, B.H.; Getlinger, M.J.; Goyal, N.V.; Alekel, L.; Hasler, C.M.; Juma, S.; Drum, M.L.; Hollis, B.W. & Kukreja, S.C. (1998b). Role of soy protein with normal or reduced isoflavone content in reversing bone loss induced by ovarian hormone deficiency in rats. *Am J Clin Nutr*, Vol. 68, No. 6 Suppl, (Dec 1998b), pp. 1358S-1363S

Arjmandi, B.H.; Khalil, D.A.; Smith, B.J.; Lucas, E.A.; Juma, S.; Payton, M.E. & Wild, R.A. (2003). Soy protein has a greater effect on bone in postmenopausal women not on hormone replacement therapy, as evidenced by reducing bone resorption and urinary calcium excretion. *J Clin Endocrinol Metab*, Vol. 88, No. 3, (Mar 2003), pp. 1048-1054

Arjmandi, B.H.; Lucas, E.A.; Khalil, D.A.; Devareddy, L.; Smith, B.J.; McDonald, J.; Arquitt, A.B.; Payton, M.E. & Mason, C. (2005). One year soy protein supplementation has positive effects on bone formation markers but not bone density in postmenopausal women. *Nutr J*, Vol. 4, No. 2005), pp. 8

Arnett, T.R. (2008). Extracellular pH regulates bone cell function. *J Nutr*, Vol. 138, No. 2, (Feb 2008), pp. 415S-418S

Ballard, T.L.; Clapper, J.A.; Specker, B.L.; Binkley, T.L. & Vukovich, M.D. (2005). Effect of protein supplementation during a 6-mo strength and conditioning program on insulin-like growth factor I and markers of bone turnover in young adults. *Am J Clin Nutr*, Vol. 81, No. 6, (Jun 2005), pp. 1442-1448

Barzel, U.S. & Massey, L.K. (1998). Excess dietary protein can adversely affect bone. *J Nutr*, Vol. 128, No. 6, (Jun 1998), pp. 1051-1053

Beasley, J.M.; Ichikawa, L.E.; Ange, B.A.; Spangler, L.; LaCroix, A.Z.; Ott, S.M. & Scholes, D. (2010). Is protein intake associated with bone mineral density in young women? *Am J Clin Nutr*, Vol. 91, No. 5, (May 2010), pp. 1311-1316

Bharadwaj, S.; Naidu, A.G.; Betageri, G.V.; Prasadarao, N.V. & Naidu, A.S. (2009). Milk ribonuclease-enriched lactoferrin induces positive effects on bone turnover markers in postmenopausal women. *Osteoporos Int*, Vol. 20, No. 9, (Sep 2009), pp. 1603-1611

Blais, A.; Malet, A.; Mikogami, T.; Martin-Rouas, C. & Tome, D. (2009). Oral bovine lactoferrin improves bone status of ovariectomized mice. *Am J Physiol Endocrinol Metab*, Vol. 296, No. 6, (Jun 2009), pp. E1281-1288

Bonjour, J.P. (2005). Dietary protein: an essential nutrient for bone health. *J Am Coll Nutr*, Vol. 24, No. 6 Suppl, (Dec 2005), pp. 526S-536S

Bonjour, J.P.; Ammann, P.; Chevalley, T. & Rizzoli, R. (2001). Protein intake and bone growth. *Can J Appl Physiol*, Vol. 26 Suppl, No. 2001), pp. S153-166

Bos, K.J.; Rucklidge, G.J.; Dunbar, B. & Robins, S.P. (1999). Primary structure of the helical domain of porcine collagen X. *Matrix Biol*, Vol. 18, No. 2, (Apr 1999), pp. 149-153

Bouxsein, M.L. (2011). Bone structure and fracture risk: do they go arm in arm? *J Bone Miner Res*, Vol. 26, No. 7, (Jul 2011), pp. 1389-1391

Bouxsein, M.L. & Seeman, E. (2009). Quantifying the material and structural determinants of bone strength. *Best Pract Res Clin Rheumatol*, Vol. 23, No. 6, (Dec 2009), pp. 741-753

Burr, D.B. (2002). The contribution of the organic matrix to bone's material properties. *Bone*, Vol. 31, No. 1, (Jul 2002), pp. 8-11

Canaff, L.; Petit, J.L.; Kisiel, M.; Watson, P.H.; Gascon-Barre, M. & Hendy, G.N. (2001). Extracellular calcium-sensing receptor is expressed in rat hepatocytes. coupling to intracellular calcium mobilization and stimulation of bile flow. *J Biol Chem*, Vol. 276, No. 6, (Feb 9 2001), pp. 4070-4079

Cao, J.J.; Johnson, L.K. & Hunt, J.R. (2011). A diet high in meat protein and potential renal acid load increases fractional calcium absorption and urinary calcium excretion without affecting markers of bone resorption or formation in postmenopausal women. *J Nutr*, Vol. 141, No. 3, (Mar 2011), pp. 391-397

Ceglia, L.; Harris, S.S.; Abrams, S.A.; Rasmussen, H.M.; Dallal, G.E. & Dawson-Hughes, B. (2009). Potassium bicarbonate attenuates the urinary nitrogen excretion that accompanies an increase in dietary protein and may promote calcium absorption. *J Clin Endocrinol Metab*, Vol. 94, No. 2, (Feb 2009), pp. 645-653

Chen, Z.; Zheng, W.; Custer, L.J.; Dai, Q.; Shu, X.O.; Jin, F. & Franke, A.A. (1999). Usual dietary consumption of soy foods and its correlation with the excretion rate of isoflavonoids in overnight urine samples among Chinese women in Shanghai. *Nutr Cancer*, Vol. 33, No. 1, 1999), pp. 82-87

Chevalley, T.; Bonjour, J.P.; Ferrari, S. & Rizzoli, R. (2008). High-protein intake enhances the positive impact of physical activity on BMC in prepubertal boys. *J Bone Miner Res*, Vol. 23, No. 1, (Jan 2008), pp. 131-142

Chevalley, T.; Hoffmeyer, P.; Bonjour, J.P. & Rizzoli, R. (2010). Early serum IGF-I response to oral protein supplements in elderly women with a recent hip fracture. *Clin Nutr*, Vol. 29, No. 1, (Feb 2010), pp. 78-83

Chiechi, L.M.; Secreto, G.; D'Amore, M.; Fanelli, M.; Venturelli, E.; Cantatore, F.; Valerio, T.; Laselva, G. & Loizzi, P. (2002). Efficacy of a soy rich diet in preventing postmenopausal osteoporosis: the Menfis randomized trial. *Maturitas*, Vol. 42, No. 4, (Aug 30 2002), pp. 295-300

Conigrave, A.D. & Brown, E.M. (2006). Taste receptors in the gastrointestinal tract. II. L-amino acid sensing by calcium-sensing receptors: implications for GI physiology. *Am J Physiol Gastrointest Liver Physiol*, Vol. 291, No. 5, (Nov 2006), pp. G753-761

Conigrave, A.D.; Brown, E.M. & Rizzoli, R. (2008). Dietary protein and bone health: roles of amino acid-sensing receptors in the control of calcium metabolism and bone homeostasis. *Annu Rev Nutr*, Vol. 28, No. 2008), pp. 131-155

Conigrave, A.D.; Quinn, S.J. & Brown, E.M. (2000). L-amino acid sensing by the extracellular Ca2+-sensing receptor. *Proc Natl Acad Sci U S A*, Vol. 97, No. 9, (Apr 25 2000), pp. 4814-4819

Cornish, J. (2004). Lactoferrin promotes bone growth. *Biometals*, Vol. 17, No. 3, (Jun 2004), pp. 331-335

Cornish, J.; Callon, K.E.; Naot, D.; Palmano, K.P.; Banovic, T.; Bava, U.; Watson, M.; Lin, J.M.; Tong, P.C.; Chen, Q.; Chan, V.A.; Reid, H.E.; Fazzalari, N.; Baker, H.M.; Baker, E.N.; Haggarty, N.W.; Grey, A.B. & Reid, I.R. (2004). Lactoferrin is a potent regulator of bone cell activity and increases bone formation in vivo. *Endocrinology*, Vol. 145, No. 9, (Sep 2004), pp. 4366-4374

Currey, J. (2001). Sacrificial bonds heal bone. *Nature*, Vol. 414, No. 6865, (Dec 13 2001), pp. 699

Dalais, F.S.; Rice, G.E.; Wahlqvist, M.L.; Grehan, M.; Murkies, A.L.; Medley, G.; Ayton, R. & Strauss, B.J. (1998). Effects of dietary phytoestrogens in postmenopausal women. *Climacteric*, Vol. 1, No. 2, (Jun 1998), pp. 124-129

Dargent-Molina, P.; Sabia, S.; Touvier, M.; Kesse, E.; Breart, G.; Clavel-Chapelon, F. & Boutron-Ruault, M.C. (2008). Proteins, dietary acid load, and calcium and risk of postmenopausal fractures in the E3N French women prospective study. *J Bone Miner Res*, Vol. 23, No. 12, (Dec 2008), pp. 1915-1922

Darling, A.L.; Millward, D.J.; Torgerson, D.J.; Hewitt, C.E. & Lanham-New, S.A. (2009). Dietary protein and bone health: a systematic review and meta-analysis. *Am J Clin Nutr*, Vol. 90, No. 6, (Dec 2009), pp. 1674-1692

Dawson-Hughes, B. & Harris, S.S. (2002). Calcium intake influences the association of protein intake with rates of bone loss in elderly men and women. *Am J Clin Nutr*, Vol. 75, No. 4, (Apr 2002), pp. 773-779

Dawson-Hughes, B.; Harris, S.S.; Palermo, N.J.; Castaneda-Sceppa, C.; Rasmussen, H.M. & Dallal, G.E. (2009). Treatment with potassium bicarbonate lowers calcium excretion and bone resorption in older men and women. *J Clin Endocrinol Metab*, Vol. 94, No. 1, (Jan 2009), pp. 96-102

Dawson-Hughes, B.; Harris, S.S.; Rasmussen, H.; Song, L. & Dallal, G.E. (2004). Effect of dietary protein supplements on calcium excretion in healthy older men and women. *J Clin Endocrinol Metab*, Vol. 89, No. 3, (Mar 2004), pp. 1169-1173

Dawson-Hughes, B.; Harris, S.S.; Rasmussen, H.M. & Dallal, G.E. (2007). Comparative effects of oral aromatic and branched-chain amino acids on urine calcium excretion in humans. *Osteoporos Int*, Vol. 18, No. 7, (Jul 2007), pp. 955-961

Debbabi, H.; Dubarry, M.; Rautureau, M. & Tome, D. (1998). Bovine lactoferrin induces both mucosal and systemic immune response in mice. *J Dairy Res*, Vol. 65, No. 2, (May 1998), pp. 283-293

Delmi, M.; Rapin, C.H.; Bengoa, J.M.; Delmas, P.D.; Vasey, H. & Bonjour, J.P. (1990). Dietary supplementation in elderly patients with fractured neck of the femur. *Lancet*, Vol. 335, No. 8696, (Apr 28 1990), pp. 1013-1016

Devine, A.; Dick, I.M.; Islam, A.F.; Dhaliwal, S.S. & Prince, R.L. (2005). Protein consumption is an important predictor of lower limb bone mass in elderly women. *Am J Clin Nutr*, Vol. 81, No. 6, (Jun 2005), pp. 1423-1428

Domrongkitchaiporn, S.; Pongskul, C.; Sirikulchayanonta, V.; Stitchantrakul, W.; Leeprasert, V.; Ongphiphadhanakul, B.; Radinahamed, P. & Rajatanavin, R. (2002). Bone histology and bone mineral density after correction of acidosis in distal renal tubular acidosis. *Kidney Int*, Vol. 62, No. 6, (Dec 2002), pp. 2160-2166

Fenton, T.R.; Eliasziw, M.; Lyon, A.W.; Tough, S.C. & Hanley, D.A. (2008). Meta-analysis of the quantity of calcium excretion associated with the net acid excretion of the modern diet under the acid-ash diet hypothesis. *Am J Clin Nutr*, Vol. 88, No. 4, (Oct 2008), pp. 1159-1166

Fenton, T.R.; Tough, S.C.; Lyon, A.W.; Eliasziw, M. & Hanley, D.A. (2011). Causal assessment of dietary acid load and bone disease: a systematic review & meta-analysis applying Hill's epidemiologic criteria for causality. *Nutr J*, Vol. 10, No. 2011), pp. 41

Feskanich, D.; Willett, W.C.; Stampfer, M.J. & Colditz, G.A. (1996). Protein consumption and bone fractures in women. *Am J Epidemiol*, Vol. 143, No. 5, (Mar 1 1996), pp. 472-479

Folman, Y. & Pope, G.S. (1969). Effect of norethisterone acetate, dimethylstilboestrol, genistein and coumestrol on uptake of [3H]oestradiol by uterus, vagina and skeletal muscle of immature mice. *J Endocrinol*, Vol. 44, No. 2, (Jun 1969), pp. 213-218

Frassetto, L.; Morris, R.C., Jr. & Sebastian, A. (2005). Long-term persistence of the urine calcium-lowering effect of potassium bicarbonate in postmenopausal women. *J Clin Endocrinol Metab*, Vol. 90, No. 2, (Feb 2005), pp. 831-834

Frassetto, L.A.; Todd, K.M.; Morris, R.C., Jr. & Sebastian, A. (1998). Estimation of net endogenous noncarbonic acid production in humans from diet potassium and protein contents. *Am J Clin Nutr*, Vol. 68, No. 3, (Sep 1998), pp. 576-583

Fujimoto, K.; Tanaka, M.; Hirao, Y.; Nagata, Y.; Mori, M.; Miyanaga, N.; Akaza, H. & Kim, W.J. (2008). Age-stratified serum levels of isoflavones and proportion of equol producers in Japanese and Korean healthy men. *Prostate Cancer Prostatic Dis*, Vol. 11, No. 3, 2008), pp. 252-257

Gahr, M.; Speer, C.P.; Damerau, B. & Sawatzki, G. (1991). Influence of lactoferrin on the function of human polymorphonuclear leukocytes and monocytes. *J Leukoc Biol*, Vol. 49, No. 5, (May 1991), pp. 427-433

Gallagher, J.C.; Satpathy, R.; Rafferty, K. & Haynatzka, V. (2004). The effect of soy protein isolate on bone metabolism. *Menopause*, Vol. 11, No. 3, (May-Jun 2004), pp. 290-298

Geusens, P.P. & Boonen, S. (2002). Osteoporosis and the growth hormone-insulin-like growth factor axis. *Horm Res*, Vol. 58 Suppl 3, No. 2002), pp. 49-55

Giannini, S.; Nobile, M.; Dalle Carbonare, L.; Lodetti, M.G.; Sella, S.; Vittadello, G.; Minicuci, N. & Crepaldi, G. (2003). Hypercalciuria is a common and important finding in postmenopausal women with osteoporosis. *Eur J Endocrinol*, Vol. 149, No. 3, (Sep 2003), pp. 209-213

Grassi, F.; Tell, G.; Robbie-Ryan, M.; Gao, Y.; Terauchi, M.; Yang, X.; Romanello, M.; Jones, D.P.; Weitzmann, M.N. & Pacifici, R. (2007). Oxidative stress causes bone loss in estrogen-deficient mice through enhanced bone marrow dendritic cell activation. *Proc Natl Acad Sci U S A*, Vol. 104, No. 38, (Sep 18 2007), pp. 15087-15092

Grey, A.; Banovic, T.; Zhu, Q.; Watson, M.; Callon, K.; Palmano, K.; Ross, J.; Naot, D.; Reid, I.R. & Cornish, J. (2004). The low-density lipoprotein receptor-related protein 1 is a mitogenic receptor for lactoferrin in osteoblastic cells. *Mol Endocrinol*, Vol. 18, No. 9, (Sep 2004), pp. 2268-2278

Grey, A.; Zhu, Q.; Watson, M.; Callon, K. & Cornish, J. (2006). Lactoferrin potently inhibits osteoblast apoptosis, via an LRP1-independent pathway. *Mol Cell Endocrinol*, Vol. 251, No. 1-2, (Jun 7 2006), pp. 96-102

Guillerminet, F.; Beaupied, H.; Fabien-Soule, V.; Tome, D.; Benhamou, C.L.; Roux, C. & Blais, A. (2010). Hydrolyzed collagen improves bone metabolism and biomechanical parameters in ovariectomized mice: an in vitro and in vivo study. *Bone*, Vol. 46, No. 3, (Mar 2010), pp. 827-834

Guillerminet, F.; Fabien-Soule, V.; Even, P.C.; Tome, D.; Benhamou, C.L.; Roux, C. & Blais, A. (2011). Hydrolyzed collagen improves bone status and prevents bone loss in ovariectomized C3H/HeN mice. *Osteoporos Int*, In Press

Guo, H.Y.; Jiang, L.; Ibrahim, S.A.; Zhang, L.; Zhang, H.; Zhang, M. & Ren, F.Z. (2009). Orally administered lactoferrin preserves bone mass and microarchitecture in ovariectomized rats. *J Nutr*, Vol. 139, No. 5, (May 2009), pp. 958-964

Hannan, M.T.; Tucker, K.L.; Dawson-Hughes, B.; Cupples, L.A.; Felson, D.T. & Kiel, D.P. (2000). Effect of dietary protein on bone loss in elderly men and women: the Framingham Osteoporosis Study. *J Bone Miner Res*, Vol. 15, No. 12, (Dec 2000), pp. 2504-2512

He, F.J.; Marciniak, M.; Carney, C.; Markandu, N.D.; Anand, V.; Fraser, W.D.; Dalton, R.N.; Kaski, J.C. & MacGregor, G.A. (2010). Effects of potassium chloride and potassium bicarbonate on endothelial function, cardiovascular risk factors, and bone turnover in mild hypertensives. *Hypertension*, Vol. 55, No. 3, (Mar 2010), pp. 681-688

Heaney, R.P. (2000). Dietary protein and phosphorus do not affect calcium absorption. *Am J Clin Nutr*, Vol. 72, No. 3, (Sep 2000), pp. 758-761

Heaney, R.P. (2007). Vitamin D endocrine physiology. *J Bone Miner Res*, Vol. 22 Suppl 2, No. (Dec 2007), pp. V25-27

Ho, S.C.; Woo, J.; Lam, S.; Chen, Y.; Sham, A. & Lau, J. (2003). Soy protein consumption and bone mass in early postmenopausal Chinese women. *Osteoporos Int*, Vol. 14, No. 10, (Oct 2003), pp. 835-842

Hunt, J.R.; Johnson, L.K. & Fariba Roughead, Z.K. (2009). Dietary protein and calcium interact to influence calcium retention: a controlled feeding study. *Am J Clin Nutr*, Vol. 89, No. 5, (May 2009), pp. 1357-1365

Ikeda, Y.; Iki, M.; Morita, A.; Kajita, E.; Kagamimori, S.; Kagawa, Y. & Yoneshima, H. (2006). Intake of fermented soybeans, natto, is associated with reduced bone loss in postmenopausal women: Japanese Population-Based Osteoporosis (JPOS) Study. *J Nutr*, Vol. 136, No. 5, (May 2006), pp. 1323-1328

Ilich, J.Z.; Brownbill, R.A. & Tamborini, L. (2003). Bone and nutrition in elderly women: protein, energy, and calcium as main determinants of bone mineral density. *Eur J Clin Nutr*, Vol. 57, No. 4, (Apr 2003), pp. 554-565

Ince, B.A.; Anderson, E.J. & Neer, R.M. (2004). Lowering dietary protein to U.S. Recommended dietary allowance levels reduces urinary calcium excretion and bone resorption in young women. *J Clin Endocrinol Metab*, Vol. 89, No. 8, (Aug 2004), pp. 3801-3807

Iwai, K.; Hasegawa, T.; Taguchi, Y.; Morimatsu, F.; Sato, K.; Nakamura, Y.; Higashi, A.; Kido, Y.; Nakabo, Y. & Ohtsuki, K. (2005). Identification of food-derived collagen peptides in human blood after oral ingestion of gelatin hydrolysates. *J Agric Food Chem*, Vol. 53, No. 16, (Aug 10 2005), pp. 6531-6536

Jackson, R.L.; Greiwe, J.S. & Schwen, R.J. (2011). Emerging evidence of the health benefits of S-equol, an estrogen receptor beta agonist. *Nutr Rev*, Vol. 69, No. 8, (Aug 2011), pp. 432-448

Jajoo, R.; Song, L.; Rasmussen, H.; Harris, S.S. & Dawson-Hughes, B. (2006). Dietary acid-base balance, bone resorption, and calcium excretion. *J Am Coll Nutr*, Vol. 25, No. 3, (Jun 2006), pp. 224-230

Kaneki, M.; Hodges, S.J.; Hosoi, T.; Fujiwara, S.; Lyons, A.; Crean, S.J.; Ishida, N.; Nakagawa, M.; Takechi, M.; Sano, Y.; Mizuno, Y.; Hoshino, S.; Miyao, M.; Inoue, S.; Horiki, K.; Shiraki, M.; Ouchi, Y. & Orimo, H. (2001). Japanese fermented soybean food as the major determinant of the large geographic difference in circulating levels of vitamin K2: possible implications for hip-fracture risk. *Nutrition*, Vol. 17, No. 4, (Apr 2001), pp. 315-321

Kerstetter, J.E. & Allen, L.H. (1990). Dietary protein increases urinary calcium. *J Nutr*, Vol. 120, No. 1, (Jan 1990), pp. 134-136

Kerstetter, J.E.; Caseria, D.M.; Mitnick, M.E.; Ellison, A.F.; Gay, L.F.; Liskov, T.A.; Carpenter, T.O. & Insogna, K.L. (1997). Increased circulating concentrations of parathyroid hormone in healthy, young women consuming a protein-restricted diet. *Am J Clin Nutr*, Vol. 66, No. 5, (Nov 1997), pp. 1188-1196

Kerstetter, J.E.; Mitnick, M.E.; Gundberg, C.M.; Caseria, D.M.; Ellison, A.F.; Carpenter, T.O. & Insogna, K.L. (1999). Changes in bone turnover in young women consuming different levels of dietary protein. *J Clin Endocrinol Metab*, Vol. 84, No. 3, (Mar 1999), pp. 1052-1055

Kerstetter, J.E.; O'Brien, K.O.; Caseria, D.M.; Wall, D.E. & Insogna, K.L. (2005). The impact of dietary protein on calcium absorption and kinetic measures of bone turnover in women. *J Clin Endocrinol Metab*, Vol. 90, No. 1, (Jan 2005), pp. 26-31

Kerstetter, J.E.; O'Brien, K.O. & Insogna, K.L. (1998). Dietary protein affects intestinal calcium absorption. *Am J Clin Nutr*, Vol. 68, No. 4, (Oct 1998), pp. 859-865

Kerstetter, J.E.; O'Brien, K.O. & Insogna, K.L. (2003). Dietary protein, calcium metabolism, and skeletal homeostasis revisited. *Am J Clin Nutr*, Vol. 78, No. 3 Suppl, (Sep 2003), pp. 584S-592S

Kerstetter, J.E.; Wall, D.E.; O'Brien, K.O.; Caseria, D.M. & Insogna, K.L. (2006). Meat and soy protein affect calcium homeostasis in healthy women. *J Nutr*, Vol. 136, No. 7, (Jul 2006), pp. 1890-1895

Khalil, D.A.; Lucas, E.A.; Juma, S.; Smith, B.J.; Payton, M.E. & Arjmandi, B.H. (2002). Soy protein supplementation increases serum insulin-like growth factor-I in young and old men but does not affect markers of bone metabolism. *J Nutr*, Vol. 132, No. 9, (Sep 2002), pp. 2605-2608

Koh, W.P.; Wu, A.H.; Wang, R.; Ang, L.W.; Heng, D.; Yuan, J.M. & Yu, M.C. (2009). Gender-specific associations between soy and risk of hip fracture in the Singapore Chinese Health Study. *Am J Epidemiol*, Vol. 170, No. 7, (Oct 1 2009), pp. 901-909

Koyama, Y.; Hirota, A.; Mori, H.; Takahara, H.; Kuwaba, K.; Kusubata, M.; Matsubara, Y.; Kasugai, S.; Itoh, M. & Irie, S. (2001). Ingestion of gelatin has differential effect on bone mineral density and body weight in protein undernutrition. *J Nutr Sci Vitaminol (Tokyo)*, Vol. 47, No. 1, (Feb 2001), pp. 84-86

Kreijkamp-Kaspers, S.; Kok, L.; Grobbee, D.E.; de Haan, E.H.; Aleman, A.; Lampe, J.W. & van der Schouw, Y.T. (2004). Effect of soy protein containing isoflavones on cognitive function, bone mineral density, and plasma lipids in postmenopausal women: a randomized controlled trial. *Jama*, Vol. 292, No. 1, (Jul 7 2004), pp. 65-74

Lampe, J.W.; Karr, S.C.; Hutchins, A.M. & Slavin, J.L. (1998). Urinary equol excretion with a soy challenge: influence of habitual diet. *Proc Soc Exp Biol Med*, Vol. 217, No. 3, (Mar 1998), pp. 335-339

Lean, J.M.; Davies, J.T.; Fuller, K.; Jagger, C.J.; Kirstein, B.; Partington, G.A.; Urry, Z.L. & Chambers, T.J. (2003). A crucial role for thiol antioxidants in estrogen-deficiency bone loss. *J Clin Invest*, Vol. 112, No. 6, (Sep 2003), pp. 915-923

Legrand, D.; Elass, E.; Carpentier, M. & Mazurier, J. (2005). Lactoferrin: a modulator of immune and inflammatory responses. *Cell Mol Life Sci*, Vol. 62, No. 22, (Nov 2005), pp. 2549-2559

Legrand, D.; Elass, E.; Carpentier, M. & Mazurier, J. (2006). Interactions of lactoferrin with cells involved in immune function. *Biochem Cell Biol*, Vol. 84, No. 3, (Jun 2006), pp. 282-290

Legrand, D.; Elass, E.; Pierce, A. & Mazurier, J. (2004). Lactoferrin and host defence: an overview of its immuno-modulating and anti-inflammatory properties. *Biometals*, Vol. 17, No. 3, (Jun 2004), pp. 225-229

Lemann, J., Jr.; Bushinsky, D.A. & Hamm, L.L. (2003). Bone buffering of acid and base in humans. *Am J Physiol Renal Physiol*, Vol. 285, No. 5, (Nov 2003), pp. F811-832

Lemann, J., Jr.; Pleuss, J.A.; Gray, R.W. & Hoffmann, R.G. (1991). Potassium administration reduces and potassium deprivation increases urinary calcium excretion in healthy adults [corrected]. *Kidney Int*, Vol. 39, No. 5, (May 1991), pp. 973-983

Lorget, F.; Clough, J.; Oliveira, M.; Daury, M.C.; Sabokbar, A. & Offord, E. (2002). Lactoferrin reduces in vitro osteoclast differentiation and resorbing activity. *Biochem Biophys Res Commun*, Vol. 296, No. 2, (Aug 16 2002), pp. 261-266

Lydeking-Olsen, E.; Beck-Jensen, J.E.; Setchell, K.D. & Holm-Jensen, T. (2004). Soymilk or progesterone for prevention of bone loss--a 2 year randomized, placebo-controlled trial. *Eur J Nutr*, Vol. 43, No. 4, (Aug 2004), pp. 246-257

Lynch, M.P.; Stein, J.L.; Stein, G.S. & Lian, J.B. (1995). The influence of type I collagen on the development and maintenance of the osteoblast phenotype in primary and passaged rat calvarial osteoblasts: modification of expression of genes supporting cell growth, adhesion, and extracellular matrix mineralization. *Exp Cell Res*, Vol. 216, No. 1, (Jan 1995), pp. 35-45

Malet, A.; Bournaud, E.; Lan, A.; Mikogami, T.; Tome, D. & Blais, A. (2011). Bovine lactoferrin improves bone status of ovariectomized mice via immune function modulation. *Bone*, Vol. 48, No. 5, (May 1 2011), pp. 1028-1035

Mallegol, J.; van Niel, G. & Heyman, M. (2005). Phenotypic and functional characterization of intestinal epithelial exosomes. *Blood Cells Mol Dis*, Vol. 35, No. 1, (Jul-Aug 2005), pp. 11-16

Mann, V.; Hobson, E.E.; Li, B.; Stewart, T.L.; Grant, S.F.; Robins, S.P.; Aspden, R.M. & Ralston, S.H. (2001). A COL1A1 Sp1 binding site polymorphism predisposes to osteoporotic fracture by affecting bone density and quality. *J Clin Invest*, Vol. 107, No. 7, (Apr 2001), pp. 899-907

Marie, P.J. (2010). The calcium-sensing receptor in bone cells: a potential therapeutic target in osteoporosis. *Bone*, Vol. 46, No. 3, (Mar 2010), pp. 571-576

Marini, H.; Minutoli, L.; Polito, F.; Bitto, A.; Altavilla, D.; Atteritano, M.; Gaudio, A.; Mazzaferro, S.; Frisina, A.; Frisina, N.; Lubrano, C.; Bonaiuto, M.; D'Anna, R.; Cannata, M.L.; Corrado, F.; Adamo, E.B.; Wilson, S. & Squadrito, F. (2007). Effects of the phytoestrogen genistein on bone metabolism in osteopenic postmenopausal women: a randomized trial. *Ann Intern Med*, Vol. 146, No. 12, (Jun 19 2007), pp. 839-847

Massey, L.K. (2003). Dietary animal and plant protein and human bone health: a whole foods approach. *J Nutr*, Vol. 133, No. 3, (Mar 2003), pp. 862S-865S

Massey, L.K. & Kynast-Gales, S.A. (2001). Diets with either beef or plant proteins reduce risk of calcium oxalate precipitation in patients with a history of calcium kidney stones. *J Am Diet Assoc*, Vol. 101, No. 3, (Mar 2001), pp. 326-331

Maurer, M.; Riesen, W.; Muser, J.; Hulter, H.N. & Krapf, R. (2003). Neutralization of Western diet inhibits bone resorption independently of K intake and reduces cortisol secretion in humans. *Am J Physiol Renal Physiol*, Vol. 284, No. 1, (Jan 2003), pp. F32-40

Mazess, R.B. & Barden, H.S. (1991). Bone density in premenopausal women: effects of age, dietary intake, physical activity, smoking, and birth-control pills. *Am J Clin Nutr*, Vol. 53, No. 1, (Jan 1991), pp. 132-142

Messina, M. (2010). Insights gained from 20 years of soy research. *J Nutr*, Vol. 140, No. 12, (Dec 2010), pp. 2289S-2295S

Metz, J.A.; Anderson, J.J. & Gallagher, P.N., Jr. (1993). Intakes of calcium, phosphorus, and protein, and physical-activity level are related to radial bone mass in young adult women. *Am J Clin Nutr*, Vol. 58, No. 4, (Oct 1993), pp. 537-542

Meyer, H.E.; Pedersen, J.I.; Loken, E.B. & Tverdal, A. (1997). Dietary factors and the incidence of hip fracture in middle-aged Norwegians. A prospective study. *Am J Epidemiol*, Vol. 145, No. 2, (Jan 15 1997), pp. 117-123

Morita, Y.; Matsuyama, H.; Serizawa, A.; Takeya, T. & Kawakami, H. (2008). Identification of angiogenin as the osteoclastic bone resorption-inhibitory factor in bovine milk. *Bone*, Vol. 42, No. 2, (Feb 2008), pp. 380-387

Morton, M.S.; Arisaka, O.; Miyake, N.; Morgan, L.D. & Evans, B.A. (2002). Phytoestrogen concentrations in serum from Japanese men and women over forty years of age. *J Nutr*, Vol. 132, No. 10, (Oct 2002), pp. 3168-3171

Munger, R.G.; Cerhan, J.R. & Chiu, B.C. (1999). Prospective study of dietary protein intake and risk of hip fracture in postmenopausal women. *Am J Clin Nutr*, Vol. 69, No. 1, (Jan 1999), pp. 147-152

Muthusami, S.; Ramachandran, I.; Muthusamy, B.; Vasudevan, G.; Prabhu, V.; Subramaniam, V.; Jagadeesan, A. & Narasimhan, S. (2005). Ovariectomy induces oxidative stress and impairs bone antioxidant system in adult rats. *Clin Chim Acta*, Vol. 360, No. 1-2, (Oct 2005), pp. 81-86

Naot, D.; Grey, A.; Reid, I.R. & Cornish, J. (2005). Lactoferrin--a novel bone growth factor. *Clin Med Res*, Vol. 3, No. 2, (May 2005), pp. 93-101

New, S.A.; MacDonald, H.M.; Campbell, M.K.; Martin, J.C.; Garton, M.J.; Robins, S.P. & Reid, D.M. (2004). Lower estimates of net endogenous non-carbonic acid production are positively associated with indexes of bone health in premenopausal and perimenopausal women. *Am J Clin Nutr*, Vol. 79, No. 1, (Jan 2004), pp. 131-138

Nijenhuis, T.; Renkema, K.Y.; Hoenderop, J.G. & Bindels, R.J. (2006). Acid-base status determines the renal expression of Ca2+ and Mg2+ transport proteins. *J Am Soc Nephrol*, Vol. 17, No. 3, (Mar 2006), pp. 617-626

Nomura, Y.; Oohashi, K.; Watanabe, M. & Kasugai, S. (2005). Increase in bone mineral density through oral administration of shark gelatin to ovariectomized rats. *Nutrition*, Vol. 21, No. 11-12, (Nov-Dec 2005), pp. 1120-1126

Oesser, S.; Adam, M.; Babel, W. & Seifert, J. (1999). Oral administration of (14)C labeled gelatin hydrolysate leads to an accumulation of radioactivity in cartilage of mice (C57/BL). *J Nutr*, Vol. 129, No. 10, (Oct 1999), pp. 1891-1895

Oh, S.M.; Lee, S.H.; Lee, B.J.; Pyo, C.W.; Yoo, N.K.; Lee, S.Y.; Kim, J. & Choi, S.Y. (2007). A distinct role of neutrophil lactoferrin in RelA/p65 phosphorylation on Ser536 by recruiting TNF receptor-associated factors to IkappaB kinase signaling complex. *J Immunol*, Vol. 179, No. 9, (Nov 1 2007), pp. 5686-5692

Ohara, H.; Matsumoto, H.; Ito, K.; Iwai, K. & Sato, K. (2007). Comparison of quantity and structures of hydroxyproline-containing peptides in human blood after oral ingestion of gelatin hydrolysates from different sources. *J Agric Food Chem*, Vol. 55, No. 4, (Feb 21 2007), pp. 1532-1535

Ohlsson, C.; Mohan, S.; Sjogren, K.; Tivesten, A.; Isgaard, J.; Isaksson, O.; Jansson, J.O. & Svensson, J. (2009). The role of liver-derived insulin-like growth factor-I. *Endocr Rev*, Vol. 30, No. 5, (Aug 2009), pp. 494-535

Oreffo, R.O.; Mundy, G.R.; Seyedin, S.M. & Bonewald, L.F. (1989). Activation of the bone-derived latent TGF beta complex by isolated osteoclasts. *Biochem Biophys Res Commun*, Vol. 158, No. 3, (Feb 15 1989), pp. 817-823

Owen, T.A.; Aronow, M.S.; Barone, L.M.; Bettencourt, B.; Stein, G.S. & Lian, J.B. (1991). Pleiotropic effects of vitamin D on osteoblast gene expression are related to the proliferative and differentiated state of the bone cell phenotype: dependency upon basal levels of gene expression, duration of exposure, and bone matrix competency in normal rat osteoblast cultures. *Endocrinology*, Vol. 128, No. 3, (Mar 1991), pp. 1496-1504

Perrini, S.; Laviola, L.; Carreira, M.C.; Cignarelli, A.; Natalicchio, A. & Giorgino, F. (2010). The GH/IGF1 axis and signaling pathways in the muscle and bone: mechanisms underlying age-related skeletal muscle wasting and osteoporosis. *J Endocrinol*, Vol. 205, No. 3, (Jun 2010), pp. 201-210

Potter, S.M.; Baum, J.A.; Teng, H.; Stillman, R.J.; Shay, N.F. & Erdman, J.W., Jr. (1998). Soy protein and isoflavones: their effects on blood lipids and bone density in postmenopausal women. *Am J Clin Nutr*, Vol. 68, No. 6 Suppl, (Dec 1998), pp. 1375S-1379S

Promislow, J.H.; Goodman-Gruen, D.; Slymen, D.J. & Barrett-Connor, E. (2002). Protein consumption and bone mineral density in the elderly : the Rancho Bernardo Study. *Am J Epidemiol*, Vol. 155, No. 7, (Apr 1 2002), pp. 636-644

Quarles, L.D.; Yohay, D.A.; Lever, L.W.; Caton, R. & Wenstrup, R.J. (1992). Distinct proliferative and differentiated stages of murine MC3T3-E1 cells in culture: an in vitro model of osteoblast development. *J Bone Miner Res*, Vol. 7, No. 6, (Jun 1992), pp. 683-692

Rahbar, A.; Larijani, B.; Nabipour, I.; Mohamadi, M.M.; Mirzaee, K. & Amiri, Z. (2009). Relationship among dietary estimates of net endogenous acid production, bone mineral density and biochemical markers of bone turnover in an Iranian general population. *Bone*, Vol. 45, No. 5, (Nov 2009), pp. 876-881

Ramshaw, J.A.; Shah, N.K. & Brodsky, B. (1998). Gly-X-Y tripeptide frequencies in collagen: a context for host-guest triple-helical peptides. *J Struct Biol*, Vol. 122, No. 1-2, 1998), pp. 86-91

Rapuri, P.B.; Gallagher, J.C. & Haynatzka, V. (2003). Protein intake: effects on bone mineral density and the rate of bone loss in elderly women. *Am J Clin Nutr*, Vol. 77, No. 6, (Jun 2003), pp. 1517-1525

Reinwald, S. & Weaver, C.M. (2010). Soy components vs. whole soy: are we betting our bones on a long shot? *J Nutr*, Vol. 140, No. 12, (Dec 2010), pp. 2312S-2317S

Roughead, Z.K.; Johnson, L.K.; Lykken, G.I. & Hunt, J.R. (2003). Controlled high meat diets do not affect calcium retention or indices of bone status in healthy postmenopausal women. *J Nutr*, Vol. 133, No. 4, (Apr 2003), pp. 1020-1026

Schurch, M.A.; Rizzoli, R.; Slosman, D.; Vadas, L.; Vergnaud, P. & Bonjour, J.P. (1998). Protein supplements increase serum insulin-like growth factor-I levels and attenuate proximal femur bone loss in patients with recent hip fracture. A randomized, double-blind, placebo-controlled trial. *Ann Intern Med*, Vol. 128, No. 10, (May 15 1998), pp. 801-809

Schwartz, A.V.; Kelsey, J.L.; Maggi, S.; Tuttleman, M.; Ho, S.C.; Jonsson, P.V.; Poor, G.; Sisson de Castro, J.A.; Xu, L.; Matkin, C.C.; Nelson, L.M. & Heyse, S.P. (1999). International variation in the incidence of hip fractures: cross-national project on osteoporosis for the World Health Organization Program for Research on Aging. *Osteoporos Int*, Vol. 9, No. 3, 1999), pp. 242-253

Seeman, E. & Delmas, P.D. (2006). Bone quality--the material and structural basis of bone strength and fragility. *N Engl J Med*, Vol. 354, No. 21, (May 25 2006), pp. 2250-2261

Sellmeyer, D.E.; Stone, K.L.; Sebastian, A. & Cummings, S.R. (2001). A high ratio of dietary animal to vegetable protein increases the rate of bone loss and the risk of fracture in postmenopausal women. Study of Osteoporotic Fractures Research Group. *Am J Clin Nutr*, Vol. 73, No. 1, (Jan 2001), pp. 118-122

Setchell, K.D.; Brown, N.M. & Lydeking-Olsen, E. (2002). The clinical importance of the metabolite equol-a clue to the effectiveness of soy and its isoflavones. *J Nutr*, Vol. 132, No. 12, (Dec 2002), pp. 3577-3584

Shanker, G.; Sorci-Thomas, M. & Adams, M.R. (1994). Estrogen modulates the expression of tumor necrosis factor alpha mRNA in phorbol ester-stimulated human monocytic THP-1 cells. *Lymphokine Cytokine Res*, Vol. 13, No. 6, (Dec 1994), pp. 377-382

Stein, G.S. & Lian, J.B. (1993). Molecular mechanisms mediating proliferation/differentiation interrelationships during progressive development of the osteoblast phenotype. *Endocr Rev*, Vol. 14, No. 4, (Aug 1993), pp. 424-442

Suda, T.; Takahashi, N.; Udagawa, N.; Jimi, E.; Gillespie, M.T. & Martin, T.J. (1999). Modulation of osteoclast differentiation and function by the new members of the tumor necrosis factor receptor and ligand families. *Endocr Rev*, Vol. 20, No. 3, (Jun 1999), pp. 345-357

Takayama, Y. & Mizumachi, K. (2008). Effect of bovine lactoferrin on extracellular matrix calcification by human osteoblast-like cells. *Biosci Biotechnol Biochem*, Vol. 72, No. 1, (Jan 2008), pp. 226-230

Takeuchi, Y.; Nakayama, K. & Matsumoto, T. (1996). Differentiation and cell surface expression of transforming growth factor-beta receptors are regulated by interaction with matrix collagen in murine osteoblastic cells. *J Biol Chem*, Vol. 271, No. 7, (Feb 16 1996), pp. 3938-3944

Takeuchi, Y.; Suzawa, M.; Kikuchi, T.; Nishida, E.; Fujita, T. & Matsumoto, T. (1997). Differentiation and transforming growth factor-beta receptor down-regulation by collagen-alpha2beta1 integrin interaction is mediated by focal adhesion kinase and its downstream signals in murine osteoblastic cells. *J Biol Chem*, Vol. 272, No. 46, (Nov 14 1997), pp. 29309-29316

Teegarden, D.; Lyle, R.M.; McCabe, G.P.; McCabe, L.D.; Proulx, W.R.; Michon, K.; Knight, A.P.; Johnston, C.C. & Weaver, C.M. (1998). Dietary calcium, protein, and phosphorus are related to bone mineral density and content in young women. *Am J Clin Nutr*, Vol. 68, No. 3, (Sep 1998), pp. 749-754

Thorpe, D.L.; Knutsen, S.F.; Beeson, W.L.; Rajaram, S. & Fraser, G.E. (2008a). Effects of meat consumption and vegetarian diet on risk of wrist fracture over 25 years in a cohort of peri- and postmenopausal women. *Public Health Nutr*, Vol. 11, No. 6, (Jun 2008a), pp. 564-572

Thorpe, M. & Evans, E.M. (2011). Dietary protein and bone health: harmonizing conflicting theories. *Nutr Rev*, Vol. 69, No. 4, (Apr 2011), pp. 215-230

Thorpe, M.; Mojtahedi, M.C.; Chapman-Novakofski, K.; McAuley, E. & Evans, E.M. (2008b). A positive association of lumbar spine bone mineral density with dietary protein is suppressed by a negative association with protein sulfur. *J Nutr*, Vol. 138, No. 1, (Jan 2008b), pp. 80-85

Tkatch, L.; Rapin, C.H.; Rizzoli, R.; Slosman, D.; Nydegger, V.; Vasey, H. & Bonjour, J.P. (1992). Benefits of oral protein supplementation in elderly patients with fracture of the proximal femur. *J Am Coll Nutr*, Vol. 11, No. 5, (Oct 1992), pp. 519-525

Turner, C.H. (2006). Bone strength: current concepts. *Ann N Y Acad Sci*, Vol. 1068, No. (Apr 2006), pp. 429-446

Uenishi, K.; Ishida, H.; Toba, Y.; Aoe, S.; Itabashi, A. & Takada, Y. (2007). Milk basic protein increases bone mineral density and improves bone metabolism in healthy young women. *Osteoporos Int*, Vol. 18, No. 3, (Mar 2007), pp. 385-390

Vatanparast, H.; Bailey, D.A.; Baxter-Jones, A.D. & Whiting, S.J. (2007). The effects of dietary protein on bone mineral mass in young adults may be modulated by adolescent calcium intake. *J Nutr*, Vol. 137, No. 12, (Dec 2007), pp. 2674-2679

Weikert, C.; Walter, D.; Hoffmann, K.; Kroke, A.; Bergmann, M.M. & Boeing, H. (2005). The relation between dietary protein, calcium and bone health in women: results from the EPIC-Potsdam cohort. *Ann Nutr Metab*, Vol. 49, No. 5, (Sep-Oct 2005), pp. 312-318

Weitzmann, M.N. & Pacifici, R. (2007). T cells: unexpected players in the bone loss induced by estrogen deficiency and in basal bone homeostasis. *Ann N Y Acad Sci*, Vol. 1116, No. (Nov 2007), pp. 360-375

Wengreen, H.J.; Munger, R.G.; West, N.A.; Cutler, D.R.; Corcoran, C.D.; Zhang, J. & Sassano, N.E. (2004). Dietary protein intake and risk of osteoporotic hip fracture in elderly residents of Utah. *J Bone Miner Res*, Vol. 19, No. 4, (Apr 2004), pp. 537-545

Whiting, S.J.; Anderson, D.J. & Weeks, S.J. (1997). Calciuric effects of protein and potassium bicarbonate but not of sodium chloride or phosphate can be detected acutely in adult women and men. *Am J Clin Nutr*, Vol. 65, No. 5, (May 1997), pp. 1465-1472

Whiting, S.J.; Boyle, J.L.; Thompson, A.; Mirwald, R.L. & Faulkner, R.A. (2002). Dietary protein, phosphorus and potassium are beneficial to bone mineral density in adult men consuming adequate dietary calcium. *J Am Coll Nutr*, Vol. 21, No. 5, (Oct 2002), pp. 402-409

Wilson, J. & Wilson, G.J. (2006). Contemporary issues in protein requirements and consumption for resistance trained athletes. *J Int Soc Sports Nutr*, Vol. 3, No. 2006), pp. 7-27

Wu, J.; Fujioka, M.; Sugimoto, K.; Mu, G. & Ishimi, Y. (2004). Assessment of effectiveness of oral administration of collagen peptide on bone metabolism in growing and mature rats. *J Bone Miner Metab*, Vol. 22, No. 6, 2004), pp. 547-553

Wynn, E.; Lanham-New, S.A.; Krieg, M.A.; Whittamore, D.R. & Burckhardt, P. (2008). Low estimates of dietary acid load are positively associated with bone ultrasound in women older than 75 years of age with a lifetime fracture. *J Nutr*, Vol. 138, No. 7, (Jul 2008), pp. 1349-1354

Xiao, G.; Wang, D.; Benson, M.D.; Karsenty, G. & Franceschi, R.T. (1998). Role of the alpha2-integrin in osteoblast-specific gene expression and activation of the Osf2 transcription factor. *J Biol Chem*, Vol. 273, No. 49, (Dec 4 1998), pp. 32988-32994

Yamamura, J.; Aoe, S.; Toba, Y.; Motouri, M.; Kawakami, H.; Kumegawa, M.; Itabashi, A. & Takada, Y. (2002). Milk basic protein (MBP) increases radial bone mineral density in healthy adult women. *Biosci Biotechnol Biochem*, Vol. 66, No. 3, (Mar 2002), pp. 702-704

Zhang, X.; Shu, X.O.; Li, H.; Yang, G.; Li, Q.; Gao, Y.T. & Zheng, W. (2005). Prospective cohort study of soy food consumption and risk of bone fracture among postmenopausal women. *Arch Intern Med*, Vol. 165, No. 16, (Sep 12 2005), pp. 1890-1895

Zhou, S.; Turgeman, G.; Harris, S.E.; Leitman, D.C.; Komm, B.S.; Bodine, P.V. & Gazit, D. (2003). Estrogens activate bone morphogenetic protein-2 gene transcription in mouse mesenchymal stem cells. *Mol Endocrinol*, Vol. 17, No. 1, (Jan 2003), pp. 56-66

Zou, Z.Y.; Lin, X.M.; Xu, X.R.; Xu, R.; Ma, L.; Li, Y. & Wang, M.F. (2009). Evaluation of milk basic protein supplementation on bone density and bone metabolism in Chinese young women. *Eur J Nutr*, Vol. 48, No. 5, (Aug 2009), pp. 301-306

Zwart, S.R.; Davis-Street, J.E.; Paddon-Jones, D.; Ferrando, A.A.; Wolfe, R.R. & Smith, S.M. (2005). Amino acid supplementation alters bone metabolism during simulated weightlessness. *J Appl Physiol*, Vol. 99, No. 1, (Jul 2005), pp. 134-140